Did You Know That . . .

Romaine lettuce has twice the fiber
and potassium of iceberg lettuce?

Strawberries can help prevent cancer
by deactivating carcinogens?

One red pepper packs more vitamin C than an orange?

Drinking one glass of wine a day can
help prevent a heart attack?

You do now, thanks to

EARL MINDELL

Earl Mindell's
FOOD AS MEDICINE

■ ■ ■

Earl Mindell, R.Ph., Ph.D.

POCKET BOOKS
New York London Toronto Sydney Singapore

The ideas, procedures, and suggestions contained in this book are not intended to replace the services of a trained health professional. All matters regarding your health require medical supervision. You should consult your physician before adopting the procedures in this book. Any applications of the treatments set forth in this book are at the reader's discretion.

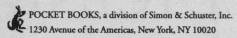 POCKET BOOKS, a division of Simon & Schuster, Inc.
1230 Avenue of the Americas, New York, NY 10020

Copyright © 1994 by Earl Mindell, R.Ph., Ph.D., and Carol Colman

Originally published in trade paperback in 1994 by Fireside

All rights reserved, including the right to reproduce
this book or portions thereof in any form whatsoever.
For information address Fireside, 1230 Avenue
of the Americas, New York, NY 10020

ISBN: 0-7432-2662-3

First Pocket Books printing June 2002

10 9 8 7 6 5 4 3 2 1

POCKET and colophon are registered trademarks of Simon & Schuster, Inc.

For information regarding special discounts for bulk purchases,
please contact Simon & Schuster Special Sales at 1-800-456-6798
or business@simonandschuster.com

Printed in the U.S.A.

Acknowledgments

I wish to express my deep and lasting appreciation to my friends and associates who have assisted me in this book, especially, Laurie Kranz Bickoff; J. Kenney, Ph.D.; Linus Pauling, Ph.D.; Harold Segal, Ph.D.; Bernard Bubman, R.Ph.; Mel Rich, R.Ph.; Sal Messineo, Pharm.D., R.Ph.; Allan Kashin, R.Ph., Ph.D.; Arnold Fox, M.D.; Gershon Lesser, M.D.; David Velkoff, M.D.; Rory Jaffee, M.D.; Donald Cruden, O.D.; Joel Strom, D.D.S., and Nathan Sperling, D.D.S. I would like to thank Kate Alfriend of the U.S. Department of Agriculture Office Public Affairs and Alegria B. Caragay of the consulting firm of Arthur D. Little for providing me with important information. A special thanks to Carol Colman Gerber and my editors, Marilyn Abraham and Sheila Curry for their help. Much thanks to my agent Richard Curtis for all his help throughout the years. I also wish to express my gratitude to the Nestle Food Museum in Vevey, Switzerland, for their research help.

Contents

Foods for Life

Food Power:
The Best
Medicine

∎ ∎ ∎

CHAPTER 1

Food ... It's Strong Medicine

In 400 B.C., Hippocrates, the "father of modern medicine," said, "Let food be your medicine and medicine be your food." After more than 2000 years, the medical establishment has finally acknowledged that he was right: food can be strong medicine.

Respectable, mainstream groups—including the National Cancer Institute and the New York Academy of Sciences—agree that nutrition can play a vital role in the prevention, treatment, and cure of a wide variety of ailments. Recent articles in distinguished professional publications, such as the *New England Journal of Medicine* and the *Journal of the American Medical Association,* report that vitamins, minerals, and other substances found in food appear to have a protective effect against certain diseases, including cancer, diabetes, high blood pressure, heart disease, and osteoporosis. They report that certain chemicals in food can retard the aging process. Indeed, many experts believe that changes in the typical American diet could extend the average life expectancy by more than ten years! Moreover, recent studies indicate that problems such as miscarriage and birth defects, once considered random events, often result from nutritional deficiencies.

As recently as a decade ago, however, few "respectable" physicians would have uttered the words "food" and "medicine" in the same breath. It would have been unthinkable to tell patients that they might be able to lower blood pressure, treat heart disease, or prevent cancer by eating certain foods. In fact, after World War II, the availability of antibiotics and other "wonder drugs" profoundly changed the way medicine was practiced in the United States. Until the middle of the twentieth century, natural remedies (herbs and food) were listed side-by-side with chemical drugs in the *U.S. Pharmacopeia,* the official listing of accepted medicines. Physicians were primarily "family physicians," who treated the "whole body"—not the specialists we have today, whose primary focus is one particular body part or system. Back then, many physicians recognized that factors such as nutrition and even stress could profoundly affect a patient's health. By the time I started pharmacy school in 1958, however, the notion that diet or life-style might somehow be related to health was considered downright unscientific. The real medicines were the pills and potions that physicians prescribed and we pharmacists dispensed. We all believed that there was nothing in nature that could possibly compete with what man could concoct in the laboratory or perform in the operating room.

In the 1950s, food quickly lost its status as a healing agent and was regarded solely as fuel for the body. Fast-food empires designed to offer a quick "fill-up" sprang up around the country selling their heavily processed, high-fat, high-sodium food. Burgers, fries, and cola became the mainstay of the American diet. Vitamins were considered necessary only to prevent the most severe deficiency diseases, such as scurvy or beriberi. When patients asked physicians about nutrition or vitamins, their questions were often dismissed with, "As long as you're eating a well-balanced diet, you have nothing to worry about." Few bothered explaining what a "well-balanced diet" was.

Those who disagreed with this approach were labeled charlatans. When the late Adelle Davis wrote that diet was a direct cause of many diseases, she was labeled a fraud. Who would have guessed that the Surgeon General of the United States would reach the same conclusion two decades later! In 1969, when Drs. Wilfred and Evan Shute, two Canadian physicians, first said that vitamin E could help prevent heart disease, they were dismissed as quacks. Today, vitamin E is routinely given to coronary bypass patients because it appears to accelerate healing and prevent new blockages from occurring. When Nobel laureate Linus Pauling began advocating the use of vitamin C as a treatment for the common cold and even speculated that it might protect against cancer, he was vilified by the medical establishment. Recent studies show that he was on the right track.

The medical community resisted the "diet-disease" link and poured its energy and money into bigger and better technology. Although hundreds of millions of dollars a year were being poured into the health care system (today, it's *hundreds of billions* of dollars), Americans were not getting much healthier.

In the 1970s, a handful of astute U.S. researchers began to question why, despite our wealth and "superior" medical knowledge, U.S. cancer and heart disease rates were high, particularly when compared with many other less-"advanced" countries around the world. They began looking for clues in "unscientific" factors such as nutrition and life-style. A pattern began to emerge: Studies showed that people who lived in less-affluent countries where the diet was rich in fruits, vegetables, and grains appeared to have protection against cancer and heart disease. Those who lived in wealthy countries where "meat and potatoes" were standard fare and other vegetables were used as garnishes (if at all) appeared to be vulnerable to these diseases. Many members of the medical establishment were quick to dismiss these findings as "coincidental" or evidence that some groups must be "genetically" prone to develop certain diseases, while others were immune. Fortunately, more thoughtful scientists took a closer look at the findings. They noticed one obvious difference: many of the "protector" foods were high in fiber and low in fat, just the opposite of the typical American diet. They concluded, quite correctly, that a high-fat, low-fiber diet must somehow increase the odds of developing heart disease and certain forms of cancer.

These pioneers also reasoned that if eating a diet rich in plant foods resulted in a lower rate of cancer or heart disease, some ingredient within these foods—vitamins, minerals, or other chemicals—might offer special protection. In laboratories throughout the world, scientists began to isolate particular chemicals in fruits and vegetables. They found that many of these "protector" foods were rich in vitamins such as beta-carotene (the plant form of vitamin A), vitamins C and E, and minerals such as selenium and potassium. They also noticed that people who consumed low levels of these key vitamins and minerals appeared to be at much higher risk of developing certain diseases.

Researchers probed further and found a wide array of other compounds in plant food, which they named phytochemicals. They tested many of these phytochemicals on animals or isolated cells to determine what, if any, role they might play in helping to prevent disease. Some of their startling discoveries were:

- ◆ Coumarins, found in plant food including parsley, licorice, and citrus fruits, are natural "blood thinners" which may prevent blood clots.
- ◆ Indoles, found in cruciferous vegetables (cabbage, broccoli, Brussels sprouts), may help to prevent breast cancer by blocking the action of potent estrogens that trigger the growth of tumors.
- ◆ Ellagic acid, found in cherries, grapes and strawberries, may deactivate carcinogens which, if left to their devices, would cause cancerous growths.
- ◆ Phytates, found in cereal grains, may deactivate steroidal compounds that promote tumors.
- ◆ Pectins, a form of soluble fiber found in apples and grapefruits, can help reduce cholesterol and may protect against diabetes.
- ◆ Genistein, a compound found in the urine of people who eat soy-based foods, appears to block the growth of new capillaries that supply blood to tumors.

The work of these researchers has led even the most skeptical members of the medical community to acknowledge that many of the diseases that plague modern men and women may actually be a result of micronutrient deficiencies—that is, a shortage of vitamins, minerals, and other biologically active substances—most of which are available in food. Not just any food, but the right food. And unfortunately, in foods that are most lacking in the American diet.

According to the National Cancer Institute, fewer than 25 percent of all Americans are actually eating the foods they should to fully protect themselves against cancer and heart disease and other common ailments. Here's the result.

◆ 1 out of 3 Americans will get cancer sometime in their lifetime, and in the twenty-first century, that figure is expected to rise to 1 out of 2.

◆ 1 out of 2 Americans will develop some form of heart disease.

◆ Breast cancer is a virtual epidemic, affecting 1 out of 9 women, with no end in sight.

◆ Among men over 50, 1 out of 11 will get prostate cancer.

◆ 15 to 20 million Americans over 45 will suffer from osteoporosis, which often leads to severe fractures and even death.

◆ 14 million Americans suffer from some form of diabetes, which greatly increases their risk of having a heart attack.

As grim as these statistics are, there are some rays of hope. According to the National Cancer Society, around 35 percent of all cancers may be related to poor diet. If we change our eating habits, we can reduce our risk of developing cancer by more than one third. In fact, many experts believe that 35 percent is actually a conservative estimate, and the number may be as high as 50 percent. The diet link may be even stronger for heart disease, the number-one killer of both men and women. In addition, other ailments, from diabetes to osteoporosis to high blood pressure, may be prevented or controlled through proper nutrition.

How Food Works

Before you can understand how the right foods can protect against various diseases, and the wrong foods may actually promote them, you need to understand how the body uses food. Here's a very abbreviated description of what happens to food in your body.

Every morsel of food you eat undergoes a complex process called digestion. It begins in the mouth, where the food is mixed with an enzyme in saliva that begins breaking it down into simple sugars. The masticated food is then swallowed and enters the esophagus, or gullet, where it is propelled through the digestive tract to the stomach. In the stomach, the food is further broken down by various enzymes and hydrochloric acid. Within a short time, the food moves on to the small intestine, which absorbs the available nutrients. From the small intestine, the food moves on to the large intestine, or colon, where it is dehydrated and forms a semisolid waste product. It takes roughly 12 to 14 hours for food to work its way through the intestinal maze until what is left of it is eliminated as feces.

The purpose of digestion is to break food down into components that can be used by the millions of cells in the body. Protein, carbohydrates, and fats provide the energy to fuel just about every body function, from breathing to thinking to walking. Vitamins work with enzymes, proteins produced by the liver, to help metabolize the nutrients from food and convert them into energy.

During the course of a given day, our bodies are exposed to many carcinogens, that is, chemicals that can promote cancer. Sometimes these chemicals are in our food—for example, the process of cooking meat can create compounds that are known carcinogens. Aflatoxin, a particularly potent carcinogen linked to liver cancer, is produced by a fungus that can grow on peanuts and other fruits and vegetables. Pollutants commonly found in the air we breathe or in our water supply may be carcinogenic. Chemicals that we use on the job may cause mutations, or changes in cells that can trigger cancer.

There are several ways that a carcinogen can do its dirty work. It can "initiate" cancer by inflicting damage on a cell, leaving the cell ripe for cancerous growth under the right circumstances. In some cases, a carcinogen can be a cancer "promoter"—it will find already vulnerable cells and turn them into cancerous ones.

Many vitamins, minerals, and other chemicals found in food may protect against cancer by promoting the production of enzymes that help to block the action of carcinogens. In some cases, a "protector" may deactivate compounds within the body that may trigger cancer. Some "protectors" are antioxidants. They prevent the formation of unstable oxygen molecules called "free radicals," which can destroy normal cells. If we don't have enough of these "protectors," then carcinogens may be allowed to run amok throughout the body.

"Protectors" do a lot more than protect against cancer. Some mediate the biochemical chain of events that produces the kind of inflammatory response that triggers conditions such as arthritis, psoriasis, and lupus. Others help the body maintain normal blood sugar levels, which can help prevent diabetes, and still others help the body better utilize the vitamins and minerals that are essential for strong bones, normal blood pressure and heart function. Some "protectors" help to strengthen the immune system, giving the body the ammunition it needs to fight its own battles.

Once you understand the valuable roles that "protectors" play in keeping us healthy, it will give you a new appreciation of the power of food.

The Future Is Bright

Within the next decade, there will be an explosion in information and interest in "food medicines." Studies involving human subjects will further explore the possible healing power of food, which I believe will greatly enhance our ability to prevent and treat many diseases. In the United States, the National Cancer Institute's Diet and Cancer Branch is in the midst of an ambitious program to study the chemo-protective properties of dozens of foods that have previously been cited as potential cancer fighters. In fact, the NCI is taking this concept one step farther by studying the possibility of extracting these compounds from food to create "designer foods" that are specifically geared to treat or prevent certain diseases. Serious researchers throughout the world, from Tel Aviv to Tokyo, from UCLA to Harvard, are investigating the potential healing properties of hundreds of foods, from tofu to curry to tuna, and are coming up with some fascinating results. Groups such as the New York Academy of Sciences are holding meetings to review the latest research on the effect of vitamins and minerals.

There are still some skeptics who say that we should wait for all the studies to be completed and data analyzed before we make any changes in our eating style. I believe they are wrong—dead wrong. While we may not yet know all the answers, we know enough of them to take positive action. However, at the rate we're going, it'll be well into the twenty-first century before the studies are done and this new information actually filters down to the public, and even longer before it is incorporated into the diets of most Americans. But there are many people who don't want to wait that long, and would like to start making changes right now. Some aren't sure exactly what to do, or are bewildered by the barrage of nutrition information presented (often inaccurately or in a confusing fashion) by the media. I've written *Earl Mindell's Food as Medicine* to close that information gap. In this book, I review the latest findings on the vitamins, minerals, and other chemicals in food that can protect against various diseases. I have also compiled a list of the "Hot Hundred" foods, which includes foods that may offer the greatest protection against disease. In addition, I try to correct misconceptions about such complex issues such as fat and cholesterol, food additives, and the controversy over food irradiation. Because having the right information can be the difference between life and death, I have included an extensive Resources section where readers can get up-to-date information and advice on various related matters.

A word of caution: Food may be good medicine, but it is not a panacea. If you are under treatment for a particular problem, do not discontinue your medicine in the hopes that a particular food will work just as well. Making positive changes in your diet may reap great benefits, and there certainly have been documented cases where people were able to slow down or even reverse some medical problems through constructive changes in their life-style. However, simply throwing out your medicine before achieving the desired result is foolhardy and can be extremely dangerous. Your best bet is to consult a naturally oriented physician who is familiar with nutrition.

An Important Point
About Food vs. Vitamins

If we know that vitamins and minerals play such an important role in preventing disease, why can't we just take a vitamin pill and stop worrying about diet?

This is one of the most common misconceptions about supplements. Many people believe that they can pop a vitamin and be healthy regardless of eating habits or life-style. This just isn't true. Vitamins and minerals are important, but in order to be effective, they need to work with food; they are not the same as food. They do not provide the same nutrients as food, nor can they satisfy hunger.

Second, the right foods contain many things that vitamins and minerals do not, such as fiber, which may prevent many different forms of cancer, as well as other phytochemicals, biologically active substances that are equally important for maintaining good health.

There are times that I may recommend taking a vitamin or mineral supplement, but that in no way diminishes the importance of food.

CHAPTER 2

The Phytochemical Pharmacy: Natural "Medicines" in Food

There are literally hundreds of compounds in foods that may offer protection against various ailments. The following chapter lists some of the major chemicals that are being investigated for potential health benefits.

Acidophilus

Lactobacillus acidophilus, better known as acidophilus, is one of the "friendly" bacteria used to ferment milk into yogurt. Physicians often advise patients taking antibiotics to eat extra yogurt because antibiotics indiscriminately kill not only the "bad" bacteria that cause illness, but also the beneficial intestinal bacteria that are necessary for digestion and that keep us well. Acidophilus has also been shown to be effective against vaginal yeast and other infections caused by the fungus, Candida albicans.

Alpha-Linolenic Acid

Alpha-linolenic acid, which is abundant in flaxseed, is one of the omega-3 polyunsaturated fatty acids, similar to those found in fatty fish such as salmon and mackerel. Alpha-linolenic acid has been shown to inhibit the metabolism of another fatty acid, linoleic, which is believed to accelerate the pace at which certain types of cancer cells multiply. This "good fat" may also help reduce the risk of heart disease and arthritis.

Antioxidants

If you leave a cut-up apple in the open air, it will turn brown, but if you sprinkle a little lemon juice over it, the apple will stay white. The discoloration of the apple is caused by a process called oxidation. Lemon juice contains vitamin C, an antioxidant, which can prevent oxidative damage not only to apples but to human cells.

Although we need oxygen to survive, certain unstable forms of oxygen molecules called "free radicals" can wreak havoc on healthy cells. Left unchecked, free radicals can combine at random with components of healthy cells and interfere with normal cell growth and activity. The cellular damage caused by free radicals is believed to be responsible for initiating many different forms of cancer and premature aging.

The oxidation of LDL or "bad" cholesterol is believed to be a major cause of atherosclerosis, a narrowing of the arteries, which can impair the flow of blood throughout the body. After the LDL cholesterol is oxidized, it attracts scavenger cells known as macrophages which literally gobble up the LDLs and form "foam cells," which gather along the arterial walls, thus beginning the formation of plaque, a thick, yellowish waxy substance. Other cells rush to the "injured" site, and the plaque keeps on growing, blocking the flow of blood throughout the body. If the oxygen flow to the heart is sufficiently reduced, it will cause a heart attack. If the arteries to the brain become blocked, it can cause a stroke.

Antioxidants can prevent the formation of free radicals or, if formed, can help stop these bad oxygen molecules in their tracks, preventing them from binding with other molecules.

Major antioxidants include vitamins C and E, carotenoids such as beta-carotene and lycopene, selenium, zinc, manganese, and coenzyme glutathione, an amino acid.

Beta-Carotene

A leading member of the carotenoid family, a group of 600 or so naturally occurring compounds found in dark leafy vegetables and yellow and orange fruits and vegetables, beta-carotene is a potent antioxidant. Unlike other carotenoids, beta-carotene is unique in that it is a precursor to vitamin A, that is, it is converted into vitamin A as the body needs it. Numerous studies have shown that people who eat diets rich in beta-carotene have lower levels of many different types of cancers, including breast cancer, colon and rectal cancer. Recent studies also show that people who eat fruits and vegetables rich in beta-carotene have lower levels of coronary artery disease.

Bioflavonoids

Also known as vitamin P, this group of compounds provide the yellow and orange color in citrus fruit and, until recently, were regarded as little more than food dye. In fact, as late as

1968, the Food and Drug Administration (FDA) deemed these compounds worthless. However, medical researchers who knew better continued to explore the potential benefits of bioflavonoids, and thanks to their work, the medical establishment is now singing a different tune. Studies show that bioflavonoids are antioxidants and may help prevent the development of certain types of cancer. In addition, specific bioflavonoids perform different functions. For example, the bioflavonoid rutin has been useful in the treatment of capillary fragility and easy bruising typical of many hypertensive patients. It has also been used to treat bleeding gums. Other bioflavonoids, quercetin, hesperidin and catechin, have been shown to have antiviral activity, in test tube experiments, against the herpes I and influenza viruses. Some bioflavonoids have also been found to reduce the inflammation caused by allergic reactions. More research is needed on bioflavonoids to determine their full potential.

Capsaicin

Capsaicin, the substance that gives chili peppers their bite, is well worth biting into. A proven anti-inflammatory, capsaicin has been used to treat cluster headaches, a particularly painful type of headache. In addition, it appears to have a beneficial effect on blood fats, and has been shown to reduce both triglycerides and LDL or bad cholesterol.

Carotenoids

The carotenoid family consists of about 600 compounds naturally occurring in fruits and vegetables; many are known antioxidants. To date, only a handful have been seriously investigated for their potential health benefits. Until recently, it has been very difficult for researchers to determine serum blood levels of specific carotenoids in humans. However, new and highly sophisticated blood testing techniques now make this possible and eventually may yield important information. Carotenoids to watch: Canthaxanthin, a carotenoid found in mushrooms and used as a food coloring in some cheeses, has been shown to help prevent breast cancer in laboratory rats. Lycopene, an antioxidant which gives some fruits and vegetables their red color, may protect against certain forms of cancer. Lutein, extracted from marigolds, spinach, and kale, is now being investigated for its potential anticarcinogenic properties.

Catechins

Catechins are bioflavonoids found in green tea and berries. Several studies have suggested that catechins can reduce the risk of gastrointestinal cancers and may help fight against viral infection.

Coumarins

Found in many fruits and vegetables, including parsley, licorice, cereal grains, and citrus fruits, coumarins are nature's own blood thinners. They protect against heart disease and stroke by preventing blood clots. In addition, coumarins are also believed to deactivate certain carcinogens before they can alter a healthy cell into one that is susceptible to cancerous growth.

Cruciferous Indoles

Found in cruciferous vegetables (cabbage, broccoli, Brussels sprouts), this compound helps prevent breast cancer by inducing protective enzymes that deactivate estrogen, which is responsible for the growth of estrogen-sensitive tumors.

Ellagic Acid

Found in cherries, grapes, and strawberries, this compound counteracts synthetic and naturally occurring carcinogens, thus preventing them from turning healthy cells into cancerous ones.

Fiber

Fiber refers to food substances found in plants that are not digested and absorbed by the body. Although fiber does not provide any calories or nutrients, it performs several important jobs in the body.

There are two types of fiber: soluble and insoluble. Soluble fiber, such as pectin and plant gum, found in such foods as apple, oat bran, and broccoli, slows down the movement of food through the intestine. Many studies have shown that soluble fiber can lower cholesterol, although the exact mechanism is unknown. Researchers suspect that soluble fiber binds with bile in the intestine and is excreted in the feces. The liver compensates for the loss of bile by producing more bile salts, of which cholesterol is a necessary ingredient, thus lowering the amount of cholesterol circulating in the blood.

Insoluble fiber, found in such foods as celery, wheat bran, kidney and pinto beans, speeds up the movement of food through the intestine. It not only helps prevent constipation and digestive diseases such as diverticulosis, but is believed to help prevent colon cancer as well as other forms of cancer, including lung, breast, and cervical cancer. Major population studies have shown that people in areas where fiber is a mainstay of the diet, such as in Africa, have significantly lower levels of colon cancer than in countries such as the United States, where the diet is typically low in fiber. For example, in Dakar, Senegal, colon cancer strikes 0.6 males and 0.7 females out of every 100,000 people. Contrast this with Connecticut, where out of 100,000 people 32.3 men and 26.4 women will contract colon cancer. Scientists aren't exactly sure how fiber helps to fight cancer, but they suspect that by speeding up the movement of food through the intestine, the contact between the intestinal lining and potential carcinogens commonly found in food is reduced. Some scientists also believe that intestinal bacteria may metabolize bile acids to carcinogenic products. Dietary fiber seems to bind to the bile acids and perhaps to other toxic products, dilute them, and literally push them out of the body. In addition, foods high in fiber tend to be low in fat and rich in vitamins and minerals, which all help to reduce the risk of cancer.

On average, Americans eat about half the 20 to 40 grams of fiber a day that is recommended by the American Cancer Society, the American Heart Association, and nearly every other major health organization. Although fiber is extremely good for you, there is the possibility of too much of a good thing. Excess amounts of fiber can interfere with absorption of calcium, iron, and other vital nutrients, so don't overdo your fiber consumption.

Genistein

This compound, found in the urine of people who eat soy-based products, such as tofu and miso soup, blocks the growth of new capillaries that supply blood to some tumors.

Researchers speculate that genistein may be responsible for the low rate of certain forms of cancer among the Japanese, who eat a diet rich in soy foods.

Glutathione

Glutathione is a combination of three amino acids, glutamate, glycine and cysteine—I call it the "triple-threat amino acid." It is a potent antioxidant that deactivates free radicals which can speed up the aging process. Some researchers say it is the most potent anticarcinogen in the body. It has also been used to help in the treatment of allergies, cataracts, diabetes, hypoglycemia, and arthritis, as well as in the prevention of the harmful side effects of high-dose radiation therapy and chemotherapy. If you are a smoker or alcohol drinker, this amino acid is for you because it helps protect your body from these poisons. Every cell can make glutathione from its components, which are found in fruits, vegetables, and raw meat (cooking can dissipate these components).

Glycyrrhetinic acid

A flavoring agent found in licorice, glycyrrhetinic acid has been shown to reduce tumors in mice, and is being investigated by the Japanese as a possible cancer treatment.

Isoflavones

Found in legumes, such as kidney beans, peas, lentils and peanuts, these compounds block estrogen receptors, thus preventing the growth of an estrogen-dependent tumor cell, the kind of cell prevalent in breast cancer. Isoflavones also deactivate estrogen before it can trigger the growth of cancerous cells.

Lignans

The flax plant is rich in compounds called lignans, which have been shown to reduce the growth of both precancerous and cancerous cells in the breast and colons of laboratory rats. Lignans are believed to deactivate potent estrogens that can stimulate tumor growth—they may turn out to be an important weapon against breast cancer. Lignans also prevent free radicals from damaging normal cells, making them susceptible to cancerous growth.

Limonene

Limonene, a constituent of citrus oil, has been found to significantly reduce the growth of mammary tumors in laboratory rats. Even better, researchers reported that this compound inhibited the formation of additional tumors in rats.

Lycopene

A member of the carotenoid family, lycopene is found in foods such as tomatoes, ruby red grapefruits, and red peppers. A recent study of 102 women with cervical cancer showed an inverse relationship between blood levels of lycopene and cervical cancer. In other words, women with low levels of lycopene are more likely to develop cervical cancer than those with high levels. Other studies have observed lower than normal levels of serum lycopene in people who develop bladder and pancreatic cancer. Researchers are not sure how lycopene protects against cancer, although they suspect that its cancer-fighting ability may be due to its antioxidant properties.

Monoterpenes

These compounds are potent antioxidants, which protect against heart disease and cancer. They are found in fruits and vegetables such as parsley, carrots, broccoli, cabbage, eggplant, cucumbers, citrus fruits, mint, and basil.

Omega-3 Fatty Acids

Omega-3 refers to two types of polyunsaturated fatty acids: docosahexaenoic acid (DHA) and eicosapentaenoic acid (EPA). Omega-3s are found primarily in marine plant life called phytoplankton and on land in flaxseed. Fish such as salmon, halibut, albacore tuna, bass, sardines, and mackerel that feed on omega-3 rich plants are primary sources of omega-3 for humans. Omega-3s offer many benefits. First, they protect against heart disease. Studies show that these fatty acids lower cholesterol and, combined with a diet reduced in saturated fats, can also reduce LDL or "bad" cholesterol as well as blood triglycerides. Omega-3s are also natural blood thinners, which prevent blood clots that can lead to heart attack or stroke. Omega-3s also protect against certain forms of cancer. Animal studies show that they can decrease the number and size of tumors. They are also anti-inflammatory and are useful in the treatment of arthritis.

Pectin

An apple a day . . . Pectin, a form of soluble fiber found in foods such as apples and the pulpy portion of grapefruit, reduces cholesterol and helps prevent heart disease. Recent research suggests that chemically altered pectin, specifically from citrus fruits, may also be potent cancer protectors. Although scientists are not sure of the exact mechanism, they believe that this chemically altered pectin may prevent malignant cancer cells from clumping together, which promotes metastases. From this research, scientists hope to develop special foods containing this special form of pectin.

Phenolic Acids

Phenolic acids or phenols, found in many foods, including garlic, flaxseed, soybean, green tea, and citrus, are antioxidants, which help prevent free-radical damage to normal cells. Phenolics also neutralize carcinogens like nitrosamines, formed in the stomach when nitrates from food combine with certain naturally occurring enzymes. They also promote the production of gluthathione, an amino acid that is believed to be the body's most potent detoxifier.

Phytates

Found in soybeans and cereal grains, these compounds deactivate steroidal hormones that promote tumors. However, an excessive amount of phytates may interfere with the absorption of minerals such as calcium.

Polyacetylenes

Bugs Bunny was right! Found in umbelliferous vegetables (carrots, celery, parsnips), these compounds mediate certain chemicals in the body called prostaglandins which can contribute to tumor growth. They also destroy benzopyrene, a particularly lethal carcinogen.

Protease Inhibitors

Western diets tend to be high in protein, and although our bodies need protein to function normally, too much protein may promote the growth of certain types of cancer. Protease inhibitors prevent protein from being digested by blocking the action of the enzymes chymotrypsin and trypsin. Studies show that protease inhibitors can prevent the conversion of normal cells to malignant ones in the earliest stages of cancer. Foods such as soybeans, kidney beans, chick peas, tofu, and whole grains such as flax and oats contain protease inhibitors.

Psoralens

Psoralens are compounds that can make skin more sensitive to sunlight and are in such fruits and vegetables as celery, lettuce, lemons, and limes. Synthetic psoralens (applied on the skin or taken orally) may be prescribed for people with skin disorders such as psoriasis who require special sunlamp therapy. Psoralens may be useful in the treatment of lymphoma.

Quercetin

Quercetin, a bioflavonoid and antioxidant, may have antiviral properties when combined with vitamin C. Quercetin has been shown to deactivate several potent carcinogens and tumor promoters. Good sources include red and yellow onions and shallots.

Quinones

Found primarily in rosemary, these compounds inhibit carcinogens, which helps protect against cancer.

Resveratrol

This compound, found in wine and Concord grape juice, has been shown to prevent coronary artery disease (atherosclerosis) in animals and possibly in humans too.

Retinoids

This group of similar compounds, including vitamin A, has been shown to have a protective effect against certain types of cancer, including lung cancer and oral cavity cancer. Retinoids are found in foods of animal origin, including liver, egg yolk, milk, and butter.

Sterols

Sterols are compounds that are found in cucumbers, especially in their skin, which has been shown to lower cholesterol.

Sulfides

Found in garlic and cruciferous vegetables, studies show that these compounds deactivate steroidal hormones that promote the growth of tumors and also inhibit carcinogens and enzymes that can cause cancer. Sulfides are also believed to help reduce blood pressure and prevent the formation of blood clots, which can cause heart attack and stroke.

Sulforaphane

Found in broccoli, Brussels sprouts, kale, cauliflower, and green onions, this compound enhances the work of enzymes that block carcinogens from damaging healthy cells. Researchers at Johns Hopkins who identified and synthesized sulforaphane believe that it has the potential to become a major weapon in the arsenal against cancer.

Triterpenoids

Found in licorice root and citrus fruit and in lesser quantities in other foods such as cereal grains and cruciferous vegetables, triterpenoids give flavors and odors to food. These compounds may also protect against cancer by deactivating steroidal hormones that promote tumor growth as well as by slowing down rapidly dividing cells, which is typical of cancer cells.

Designer Foods

Experts predict that within the next decade, supermarket shelves will be filled with specially designed "medicinal foods" (also called "nutri-ceuticals"), fortified with phytochemicals that may protect against various diseases. You could find yourself strolling down the supermarket aisle and asking a clerk, "Can you please tell me where I can find the anticancer cereals?" His reply, "They're on Aisle 3, next to the cholesterol cutters and antiosteoporosis bone builders."

The National Cancer Institute is leading the way with its much publicized Experimental Foods Project, a five-year program to study the viability of creating special foods that are enriched with naturally occurring anticancer substances. The NCI is looking at several foods that appear to have the most cancer protection potential, such as broccoli, garlic, parsley, and carrots. Researchers are hoping to isolate the "protector" compounds in these foods and test them for safety and efficacy in higher doses. Before these foods are marketed, however, there are many questions that need to be addressed. For example, if a small amount of indoles from broccoli protects against breast cancer, would a higher dose offer even more protection? Could higher doses of phytochemicals be toxic? What are the right combinations of vitamins, minerals, and phytochemicals?

Several food manufacturers are already marketing "medicinal foods" of sorts. For example, today you can choose between regular orange juice and orange juice that is fortified with calcium, which may help to prevent osteoporosis. Among the rows of breakfast cereals, you can select one made from psyllium flakes, which may lower cholesterol and prevent colon cancer. In years to come, you may see other fortified foods designed to prevent or treat such common ailments as arthritis, diabetes, many different forms of cancer, atherosclerosis, infertility, and even some for PMS and menopause.

CHAPTER 3

The Healing Power of Vitamins and Minerals: From A to Zinc

Vitamins and minerals found in food play a critical role in maintaining health. The latest research on vitamins and minerals has revealed many uses for them as "preventive medicine."

What Are Vitamins?

Vitamins are organic substances that are essential for life. In most cases, they are not produced by the body (or are not produced in sufficient quantities) and must be obtained from food or supplements. Vitamins are required for nearly every bodily process. Without the help of vitamins, we couldn't digest our food, fight off infection, or manufacture new cells.

Vitamins are called micronutrients because the amounts that are required for normal functioning are minuscule. However, even a seemingly minor deficiency of just one key vitamin may result in serious consequences.

Nutrients that provide us with energy—protein, carbohydrates, and fat—are called macronutrients and are ingested in much greater quantities. Without vitamins, however, these macronutrients could not be digested and broken down into energy.

Vitamins are usually divided into two categories: fat- or oil-soluble and water-soluble. Vitamins A, D, E, and K are fat-soluble, which means that they require an adequate supply of fat and minerals to be absorbed adequately in the digestive system. Fat-soluble vitamins are stored in the liver. The remaining vitamins are water-soluble: any excess is excreted in urine. Since water-soluble vitamins are not stored in the body, they need to be replenished daily.

Most water-soluble vitamins are measured in milligrams (mg) and micrograms (mcg). Fat-soluble vitamins are usually measured in international units (IU). However, vitamin A is sometimes measured in retinol equivalents (RE). One RE is roughly five times more than 1 IU.

Throughout this book, I may refer to the RDA (Recommended Daily Allowance) for a specific vitamin or mineral. The RDA is set by the Food and Nutrition Board of the National Academy of Sciences. The RDA is merely a rough estimate of the minimum amount of the vitamin or mineral required for normal growth in children and to prevent nutritional deficiencies in healthy adults. (The USRDA, set by the Food and Drug Administration, FDA, is used as a legal standard for food labeling and is similar to the RDA.) The RDA is not meant to be an optimal intake. In my opinion, and in the opinion of many other experts, the RDAs are woefully inadequate and do not take into account the latest findings on the importance of vitamins and minerals.

In most cases, vitamins and minerals can be taken at much higher doses than the RDA without any problem. However, some vitamins and minerals can be toxic at extremely high doses. On rare occasion, a problem can arise if someone indiscriminately pops pill after pill without paying attention to appropriate dose. If you take supplements, be sure to read the section "The Right Amount" listed for each vitamin and mineral.

I would not worry about overdosing on vitamins or minerals from food even if you also take supplements—in fact, most people have just the opposite problem: they are not getting enough essential nutrients from their diet.

What Are Minerals?

Minerals are naturally occurring chemical elements of which several are found in our bodies. Minerals such as calcium, phosphorus, and potassium, known as the essential minerals, are key components of our teeth, bones, blood cells, and soft tissue and are also essential for proper fluid balance and normal cell and muscle activity. Essential minerals are required in amounts from several hundred milligrams a day to 1 or more grams, as in the case of calcium, phosphorus, magnesium, sodium, potassium, and chloride. Minerals that are required in much smaller quantities are called trace minerals; they include iron, zinc, iodine, copper, manganese, fluoride, chromium, selenium, molybdenum, and cobalt (as a component of vitamin B_{12}).

The following is a list of important vitamins and minerals, and the latest information on the role they may play in preventing disease.

Vitamin A

FACTS Vitamin A plays many vital roles in the body; it is essential for healthy skin and mucous membranes. Vitamin A combines with a protein to form visual purple, the substance that enables us to see at night. Vitamin A is an immune booster: it helps promote the production of T lymphocytes, the body's first line of defense against infection. Vitamin A is particularly potent against respiratory ailments.

Vitamin A, which is fat-soluble, occurs in two forms: preformed vitamin A and provitamin A. Preformed vitamin A is actually a compound called retinol, which belongs to the retinoid family. Retinoids occur in foods of animal origin, such as liver, egg yolks, milk, and butter.

Provitamin A, or beta-carotene, is one of 600 carotenoids, a family of similar compounds of which only a handful have been closely studied. The body can convert beta-carotene into vitamin A if there is a deficiency. Carotenoids are found in dark green leafy vegetables and in yellow and orange vegetables and fruits. Good food sources include apricots, broccoli, kale, mustard greens, cantaloupe, carrots, mangoes, papaya, peaches, spinach, yellow squash, sweet potatoes, Brussels sprouts, and pumpkin.

Beta-carotene is a potent antioxidant. When beta-carotene is converted into vitamin A, it loses its antioxidant effect.

THE RIGHT AMOUNT Preformed vitamin A or retinol is measured in either international units (IU) or retinol equivalents (RE).

The RDA for preformed vitamin A is 5000 IU or 1000 RE.

Preformed vitamin A can be toxic in high doses. Do not exceed 25,000 IU on any given day.

Excess preformed vitamin A can cause birth defects; pregnant women should not take more than 5000 IU daily.

Provitamin A (beta-carotene) is rarely toxic at any level.

Beta-carotene is measured in mg, with 3 mg of beta-carotene = 5000 IU provitamin A.

The American diet is seriously deficient in beta-carotene. The average daily intake is under 2 mg: many scientists believe that for maximum protection against disease, we need 6 mg of beta-carotene daily.

POSSIBLE BENEFITS   At one time, research on vitamin A lumped beta-carotene, retinol, and other carotenoids together. Today, scientists are more careful to examine which compounds perform specific tasks within the body. We now know that beta-carotene and retinols have different yet equally important roles to play in protecting people against disease.

Cancer   Several studies strongly suggest that beta-carotene and, in some cases, vitamin A may be potent weapons against cancer. In general, population studies have showed higher rates of cancer among groups who ate less green leafy vegetables than among populations that ate more of these foods. However, specific studies show that beta-carotene may be useful against specific forms of cancer.

Oral and esophageal cancer: These types of cancer are closely linked to tobacco use and excessive alcohol intake. Some studies show that low levels of consumption of fruits and vegetables and low plasma beta-carotene levels have been noted in populations with the highest rates of oral and esophageal cancer. Vitamin A is also believed to be a potent inhibitor of tumor formation in oral cavity cancer.

Stomach cancer: Several studies show that consumption of green and yellow leafy vegetables was associated with lower levels of stomach cancer, and that lower levels of beta-carotene were found in the serum of people who subsequently developed stomach cancer.

Colon and rectal cancer: Consumption of fruits and vegetables has been associated with decreased risks of cancers of the colon and the rectum in several studies. Researchers, however, are not willing to give beta-carotene all the credit. Fruits and vegetables are also rich in other vitamins, other carotenoids, and even fiber, all of which may play a role in preventing this kind of cancer.

Bladder cancer: A handful of studies link lower levels of beta-carotene with an increased risk of bladder cancer.

Breast cancer: Recently, researchers in Buffalo, New York, studied 83 women with breast cancer and 113 well women. They found that the women with cancer had lower concentrations of plasma beta-carotene than those free of the disease.

In another study of 439 postmenopausal women in western New York State, researchers found that those with the lowest ingestion of beta-carotene had the highest risk of developing breast cancer after other factors were weighed, including family history, age of first pregnancy, etc.

Cervical cancer: Some studies suggest an inverse relationship between intake of fruits and vegetables and developing cervical cancer. One recent study by the National Cancer Institute done in Latin America, where the cervical cancer rates are among the highest in the world, suggested that a high beta-carotene intake was associated with a 32 percent lower risk of cervical cancer.

Oral cancers: Oral cavity cancers are closely linked to use of tobacco and alcohol. Animal studies have shown that beta-carotene, vitamins A and E are potent inhibitors of cancer formation, and researchers are working on human trials to determine the appropriate treatment.

Lung cancer: Researchers at Johns Hopkins School of Hygiene and Public Health compared the serum blood levels of men and women who subsequently developed lung cancer with those who did not. Based on these findings, the researchers hypothesized that low levels of serum beta-carotene appear to significantly increase the risk of squamous-cell carcinoma of the lung. (Low levels of vitamin E increase the risk of all forms of lung cancer.) Other studies suggest the protective value of beta-carotene against lung cancer may be even stronger in women.

Heart

Several studies suggest that beta-carotene is a major protector against coronary artery disease, which can lead to heart attack and stroke. An antioxidant, beta-carotene can help prevent the kind of oxidative damage of lipids that is believed to promote the formation of plaque in the arteries.

The Physicians' Health Study, directed by Charles Hennekens, M.D., of Brigham and Women's Hospital in Boston, followed 22,000 male physicians, ages 40 to 84. Out of that group, 333 men with chronic, unstable angina were given 50 mg of beta-carotene daily. Those taking beta-carotene had reduced risks of heart attack, revascularization procedures, bypass surgery, angioplasty to open clogged arteries, and cardiovascular death by an average of 49 percent.

Ongoing research in the Nurses' Health Study on 87,245 nurses indicates that roughly one serving a day of fruits or vegetables rich in beta-carotene can substantially reduce the risk of heart attack and stroke in healthy women. Women taking more than 15 to 20 milligrams a day of beta-carotene had a 40 percent reduced risk of stroke and 22 percent less risk of heart attack.

Eyes

Vitamin A is essential for the formation of visual purple, which is important for night vision. Recent studies suggest that beta-carotene may help prevent a common eye problem among the elderly: cataracts. A two-year study of nurses by researchers at Harvard University showed that women who eat lots of fruits or vegetables rich in carotenes have a 39 percent lower risk of developing severe cataracts than those with a low carotene intake. Foods such as spinach, sweet potatoes, and winter squash were the best protectors. The study yielded one big surprise: Carrots did not make it on the list!

Skin

For decades, vitamin A has been dubbed the "skin vitamin." Due to its antioxidant properties, beta-carotene has been touted as a means of preventing premature aging of the skin. In Europe, skin creams made from antioxidants such as beta-carotene and vitamin E are sold as skin rejuvenators. Synthetic derivatives of vitamin A, Retin-A and Tigason, are commonly used to treat acne and psoriasis. (Retin-A in cream form has been shown to reduce wrinkles and other outward signs of aging.) The oral forms of vitamin A used for skin problems are very potent drugs that can cause birth defects and should not be used by pregnant women.

The B-Complex Family

Vitamin B₁ (Thiamine)

FACTS Vitamin B₁, also called thiamine, is a water-soluble vitamin. It's main task is to break down carbohydrates from food and convert them into glucose, a sugar that provides the fuel needed to run the brain and nervous system. A severe thiamine deficiency can cause beriberi, which can adversely affect the normal functioning of the nervous system. People who are thiamine-starved often suffer from mental confusion as well as physical symptoms such as loss of feeling in the feet and legs and paralysis of the eye muscles.

Good food sources for vitamin B₁ include ham and pork, sunflower seeds, peanuts, and pompano fish. Many ready-to-eat cereals are fortified with thiamine. Smaller quantities of thiamine are present in green peas, Jerusalem artichoke, corn, and melon. As with other water-soluble vitamins, thiamine can be lost in cooking fluid.

THE RIGHT AMOUNT The official RDA for thiamine for adults is between 1.0 to 1.5 mg.

During pregnancy and lactation, women need 1.4 to 1.6 mg.

Women, but not men, between 19 and 50 tend to fall somewhat short of the RDA.

Several studies show that older people do not get enough thiamine in their diets.

Thiamine can be destroyed by alcohol, and thiamine deficiency is very common among alcoholics.

POSSIBLE BENEFITS

Eyes A recent study published in the *Archives of Ophthalmology* notes that people who were given multivitamins containing, among other things, thiamine are less likely to develop cataracts than those who were not.

Physical and Mental Well-Being Thiamine has been called the "morale vitamin" because of its effect on the nervous system.

People who are very active and eat a lot need more of this vitamin to help them utilize their food.

Shingles There have been scattered reports that intramuscular shots of thiamine have been successfully used to treat herpes zoster (shingles), a very painful disorder. However, this is not an accepted treatment.

Vitamin B$_2$ (Riboflavin)

FACTS Vitamin B$_2$, also called riboflavin, a water-soluble vitamin, helps the body release energy from protein, carbohydrate, and fat.

Good food sources include milk, cheese, yogurt, beef, fortified breads and cereals, and green vegetables such as broccoli, turnip greens, asparagus, and spinach.

THE RIGHT AMOUNT The RDA for riboflavin is between 1.3 mg and 1.7 for adults.

People who are very active, pregnant women, and nursing mothers need more of this vitamin.

POSSIBLE BENEFITS

Cancer Many scientists suspect that low levels of riboflavin may increase the odds of developing cancer of the esophagus. They theorize that riboflavin may somehow detoxify chemicals in alcohol or chewing tobacco that promote this form of cancer.

Physical Stress Riboflavin appears to help the body cope better with stressful situations. According to a study performed by researchers at Cornell University, older women in particular seem to need more of this B vitamin. In the study, women between the ages of 50 to 57 exercised for 20 to 25 minutes daily on a stationary cycle for eight weeks. Half were given the RDA for riboflavin, half were given 150 percent of the RDA. The group that had been given only the RDA experienced a drop in riboflavin after exercising, while the group that had been given a greater amount of B_2 maintained closer to normal blood levels throughout the exercise. The researchers concluded that the need for riboflavin increased with activity. Several studies show that older people tend to fall short of the RDA for riboflavin, just at a point in their lives when their bodies may need it the most. According to *The Surgeon General's Report on Nutrition and Health,* a Boston study of older people reported that more than a third had inadequate levels of riboflavin.

PERSONAL ADVICE Riboflavin can be destroyed by light. Therefore, store fortified breads and cereals in containers that will keep out light.

Vitamin B₃ (Niacin)

FACTS Vitamin B₃, also known as niacin, niacinamide, and nicotinic acid, works with thiamine and riboflavin in the metabolism of carbohydrates and is essential for providing energy for cell tissue growth. Vitamin B₃ is water-soluble.

Good food sources are mackerel, swordfish, chicken, Cornish hen, fortified ready-to-eat cereals, lean veal, and liver. Small amounts of niacin (under 24 percent of the RDA) are present in most bread products. Niacin can be made in the body from the amino acid tryptophan, which is abundant in milk and eggs. Therefore, if your diet is rich in tryptophan, your need for outside sources of niacin is reduced.

Severe niacin deficiency will result in pellagra, a debilitating disease that starts with a reddish rash in areas exposed to the sun and a swollen tongue and quickly progresses to dementia and even death.

THE RIGHT AMOUNT The RDA for adult women is 15 mg and for adult men, 19 mg. Lactating women need 16 mg.

At least two recent studies show that many people are somewhat deficient in this vitamin. Researchers speculate that as people cut back on meat to reduce fat, they are losing a major niacin source. However, adding more grains to your diet will pick up the slack.

POSSIBLE BENEFITS

Cancer Scientists at the University of Kentucky's Markey Cancer Center have reported that niacin may play a role in cancer protection. The researchers studied the effect of niacin deficiency on animal and human cells. The niacin-deprived cells began to show signs of malignant transformation which are often a precursor of cancer. Although the exact role of niacin in preventing cancer is still unknown, based on these studies this B vitamin may be an important player in keeping the body cancer-free.

Heart Niacin supplements in very high doses—much higher than you can possibly get from food alone—have been shown to lower overall blood cholesterol and raise HDLs, the good cholesterol. High amounts of niacin, however, can cause flushing and itching, which can be quite uncomfortable. I recommend using the so-called "No Flush" niacin supplements with inositol hexanicotinate, which may help reduce some of the discomfort.

Vitamin B_6 (Pyridoxine)

FACTS This vitamin plays a critical role in metabolism of nucleic acids, helps use protein to build body tissue, and aids in the metabolism of fat. It is also necessary for the production of antibodies and red blood cells. A water-soluble vitamin, B_6 is excreted from the body eight hours after ingestion.

Good food sources include fortified instant oatmeal, fortified ready-to-eat cereals, chicken, beef liver and, to a lesser degree, other cuts of beef. Smaller amounts of B_6 (under 12 percent of the RDA) can be found in cantaloupe, cabbage, blackstrap molasses, and milk.

THE RIGHT AMOUNT The RDA is 1.6 mg for adult women and 2 mg for adult men.

As protein intake increases, so does need for B_6.

Many women do not get enough of this vitamin. According to the U.S. Department of Agriculture (USDA), the average woman consumes 70 percent of the RDA. Men do somewhat better, taking in 90 percent of the RDA for them. The elderly in particular often fall short of this vitamin and may, in fact, need somewhat more than the RDA.

POSSIBLE BENEFITS

Heart According to the Physicians' Health Study, not getting enough B_6 and folate could result in a visit to the coronary care unit. B_6 and folate help to break down homocysteine, an amino acid that appears to play a role in heart disease. Based on this study, people with the highest levels of homocysteine in their blood were three times more likely to develop heart attacks than those with lower levels. Eating lots of food rich in B_6 and folate will lower homocysteine levels, thus protecting against having a heart attack.

Immunity B_6 appears to be an immune booster, especially for the elderly. Researchers recently investigated the effect of vitamin B_6 depletion on the immune systems of eight healthy elderly people and found that those with low levels of B_6 had depressed immune systems. B_6 deficiency appears to impair interleukin-2 production and lymphocyte proliferation, two important parts of the body's defense system against unwanted intruders. The bottom line: the people who were B_6 deficient were not as well prepared to fight against infection as those with higher levels of this vitamin.

CAUTION Daily doses exceeding 2000 mg can cause serious neurological damage.

Vitamin B_{12} (Cobalamin)

FACTS Vitamin B_{12} is unique among water-soluble vitamins in two important ways. First, it is the only vitamin that also contains essential mineral elements. Second, it can be stored in the body; it can take up to three years to deplete your supply. B_{12} aids in the formation of red blood cells, in the functioning of the nervous system, and in metabolizing protein and fat.

In recent years, B_{12} supplements have been given to combat fatigue and to alleviate neurological problems among the elderly, including weakness and memory loss.

B_{12} deficiency can result in pernicious anemia, a severe life-threatening condition. B_{12} works in conjunction with another B vitamin, folacin or folic acid. Folic acid cannot be utilized without adequate amounts of B_{12}.

Good food sources of B_{12} are meat, fish, eggs, and dairy products.

THE RIGHT AMOUNT The RDA for B_{12} is 2 mcg for both adult men and women.

Strict vegetarians, who avoid dairy and eggs, may be at risk of B_{12} deficiency.

Women taking oral contraceptives and heavy drinkers may also need to increase their intake of this vitamin.

Elderly people are also at risk of not getting enough vitamin B_{12}—in fact, as many as 10 percent of all elderly people may be deficient in B_{12}. B_{12} is available in capsules, tablets, a nasal gel, and a sublingual form that dissolves under the tongue.

POSSIBLE BENEFITS

Cancer Vitamin B_{12} may help protect against smoking-induced lung cancer, according to a study reported in the *American Journal of Clinical Nutrition* in 1987. Researchers studied 73 male heavy smokers who had potentially cancerous changes in their bronchial tissue. Half the men were given folic acid and B_{12} supplements, half were given a placebo. Within four months, the group on the vitamin supplements showed fewer potentially dangerous cells than the group that was not taking the B_{12} and folic acid.

Neurological Symptoms in Elderly Many people over 60 suffer from vitamin B_{12} deficiency, which is characterized by neurological symptoms ranging from a loss of balance to mood changes, memory loss, and tingling sensations in the arms and legs. Diet is not the culprit; rather, as we age, our bodies produce less hydrochloric acid, which is essential for the utilization of B_{12}. Therefore, many older people are not getting an adequate supply of this vitamin from their food. What makes matters worse is that it's easy to dismiss B_{12} deficiency symptoms in the elderly as a natural part of the aging process; however, these symptoms should not be ignored. If someone over 60 appears confused and complains of neurological symptoms, ask him/her to talk to a physician and have the B_{12} levels checked. I've seen older people make remarkable progress on alternate sources of B_{12} (the nasal gel and the sublingual form) which bypass the stomach and are absorbed directly into the bloodstream.

Biotin

FACTS Biotin, also called enzyme R or vitamin H, is actually a member of the B-complex family. This water-soluble vitamin can be synthesized in the intestines as well as derived from food. Biotin is essential for the normal metabolism of fat and protein and for the absorption of vitamin C. This vitamin works with vitamins A, B_2, B_6, and niacin to maintain healthy skin. Biotin deficiency can result in eczema or red patchy scales on the face and hair loss.

Good food sources include fruit, nuts, brewer's yeast, beef liver, peanut butter, cauliflower, egg yolk, and whole grain foods.

THE RIGHT AMOUNT The RDA for adults is 300 mcg.

Estrogen interferes with biotin absorption; therefore, women on oral contraceptives should talk to their physicians about taking a supplement.

POSSIBLE BENEFITS

Nails Do you suffer from thin, splitting nails? There is some evidence that biotin may help unsightly nails. Swiss researchers gave 2.5 mg of biotin to 32 men and women with problem nails for up to nine months. According to the study recently published in the *Journal of the American Academy of Dermatology*, by the end of the treatment participants experienced a 25 percent increase in nail thickness.

Hair Severe biotin deficiency can cause hair loss in animals and humans, which is why biotin is sometimes touted as a "hair rejuvenator." Enthusiasts claim that it can prevent both baldness and premature graying. There is no scientific evidence supporting this claim. However, I have heard anec-dotal evidence that this vitamin can make flyaway hair more manageable.

CAUTION Raw eggs can prevent absorption of biotin by the body. Raw eggs are a potential source of salmonellae, so you shouldn't be eating them anyway.

Folacin (Folic Acid)

FACTS A member of the B family, folacin, also called folic acid or folate, has been making headlines as a potential can-cer fighter. Folic acid helps in the formation of red blood cells and genetic material in the cells.

The word *folacin* is derived from the word *foliage;* this vitamin is found in dark green leafy vegetables such as spinach and broccoli. However, other good sources include legumes—dried beans are especially high in folic acid—yeast, liver, peanuts, sunflower seeds, wheat germ, and forti-fied breakfast cereals. Banana, spinach, and orange also provide more than 25 percent of the RDA.

THE RIGHT AMOUNT The RDA for folic acid is 400 mcg or 0.4 mg.

An intake of more than 0.8 mg is not advisable because it can make it difficult to diagnose a vitamin B_{12} deficiency, which can lead to anemia and damage to the nervous system.

Women on average get only half their RDA for folic acid.

Pregnant women must have their full 0.4 mg a day (roughly the amount in 1½ cups of boiled spinach or a ½ cup of peanuts) or risk serious birth defects. If their diets fall short of this amount, they must use a supplement.

Other women who are most likely to be deficient in folic acid are those on birth control pills and heavy drinkers.

POSSIBLE BENEFITS

Birth Defects Neural tube defects, such as spina bifida and anencephaly, affect 2500 infants born in the United States each year. In spina bifida, a piece of the spinal cord protrudes from the spinal column, causing paralysis in the lower body and sometimes retardation. In anencephaly, the baby is born with an incomplete brain and cannot survive. Folic acid has long been suspected of preventing neural tube defects, but past studies have been inconclusive, until recently. The July 1991 issue of the British medical journal *Lancet* reported a well-done study of 1817 women in six countries with a previous history of neural tube births. The women were randomly assigned to four groups: one took folic acid, one took folic acid and a mixture of other vitamins, one took just the other vitamins, and the last took none. The other vitamins alone did not appear to affect the outcome of the pregnancy, but those taking folic acid were 72 percent less likely to have a neural tube defect child than those who did not take folic acid. These impressive results spurred the U.S. Public Health Service to warn women who are even *considering* getting pregnant to make sure that they get their full 0.4 mg of folic acid daily. (Don't wait until you know for sure: The closure of the neural tube occurs very early in pregnancy, before some women even know they are pregnant.)

Cancer Folic acid is believed to play a role in preventing cervical cancer, the most common form of cancer among women in developing countries. Recent studies suggest that folic acid may help to prevent this form of cancer. Researchers at the University of Alabama at Birmingham compared 294 women diagnosed with cervical dysplasia, the presence of abnormal cells in the cervix, with 170 women without abnormal cells. They found that those with the lowest levels of folic acid were five times more likely to develop cervical dysplasia than women with normal blood levels of folic acid. The researchers theorized that women with low red blood cell folate levels may be more vulnerable to HPV-16, a virus that sometimes leads to cervical cancer, than those with normal levels of this vitamin.

Colon and Rectal Cancer Recently, researchers compared the diets of people who developed colorectal cancer with the diets of people who remained cancer-free. One striking difference: those who developed colorectal cancer ate significantly less foods rich in folic acid than those who did not get cancer.

CAUTION Epileptics should consult their physicians before taking folic acid since it can interfere with anticonvulsive medications. Pregnant women should not take any vitamin supplements without first consulting with their physician or midwife.

Pantothenic Acid

FACTS Pantothenic acid, a member of the B-complex family, was discovered in 1935 by biochemist R. J. Williams, who noticed that this substance was necessary for the growth of yeast, but wasn't sure that it had any role to play in the human body. We now know that pantothenic acid, in conjunction with coenzyme A, helps convert nutrients into energy and has other important tasks to perform.

Through the years, pantothenic acid has been touted as an energy booster that can enhance athletic ability, and some people swear that it can keep hair from turning gray. More research is needed to back up these claims.

Pantethine, a metabolite of pantothenic acid, has received a great deal of publicity lately because of its ability to lower cholesterol.

Good food sources include yeast, liver, eggs, peas, peanuts and wheat germ, lean meats, and legumes.

THE RIGHT AMOUNT The RDA is 10 mg, which is easy enough to obtain from food. People who need to cut their cholesterol may be given doses up to 1000 mg daily by their physicians.

POSSIBLE BENEFITS

Cholesterol Studies show that pantethine supplements can significantly lower both cholesterol (by about 15 percent) and triglycerides (by about 30 percent) in patients with elevated blood lipid levels. High triglycerides and cholesterol increase the odds of having a heart attack or stroke.

Vitamin C (Ascorbic Acid)

FACTS Vitamin C, which is water-soluble, is essential for the formation of collagen, the substance that binds together the cells of connective tissue. Collagen is necessary for the production and growth of new cells and tissues; it also prevents viruses from penetrating the cell membrane. (Viruses can reproduce only within the cell.) Since collagen is a major component of scar tissue, it is especially important in the healing process. Vitamin C also helps in the absorption of iron.

The walls of small blood vessels are made up largely of connective tissue; therefore, bleeding is one of the most common signs of vitamin C deficiency. Scurvy, a disease that can result from a lack of vitamin C, is characterized by bleeding gums, loss of teeth caused by weakened bones, and internal bleeding, which can be very painful.

Vitamin C is also a potent antioxidant, and has also been shown to deactivate carcinogens that could promote cancerous changes in the cells.

Good food sources of vitamin C include sweet red pepper, orange juice, plantain, snow peas, pineapple juice (not chunks), strawberries, asparagus, Brussels sprouts, tangerine, tangelo, watermelon, mango, papaya, honeydew melon, kiwifruit, grapefruit, orange sections, cantaloupe, cranberry juice, apple juice containing added C, broccoli, cauliflower, kale, kohlrabi, white potatoes with skin, tomatoes, and berries.

THE RIGHT AMOUNT About half of the U.S. population get less than the RDA of 60 mg of vitamin C, even though that amount is woefully low.

Since smoking destroys vitamin C, the RDA for smokers is 100 mg; however, one study found smokers may need up to 200 mg to maintain adequate levels.

Eating five servings of fruits and vegtables daily will give you between 200 and 300 mg, which I believe is the bare minimum amount required for good health.

If you take a supplement, keep in mind that excess vitamin C can cause diarrhea, excessive urination, dry nose, and skin rashes. I recommend from 1000 to 2000 mg daily; however, if you have any unpleasant side effects, take a lower dose. Calcium ascorbate is the gentlest form of vitamin C for your stomach.

Cancer There have been scores of studies on the role of vitamin C and vitamin-C-rich foods in the fight against cancer. The vast majority of these studies confirm that vitamin C is one of the body's strongest defenses against many different forms of cancer, as outlined below.

Oral, laryngeal, and esophageal cancers: Several important, well-controlled studies found that low intake of vitamin C or fruit significantly increased the risk of oral cancers.

Lung cancer: Several studies show that people who consumed higher levels of vitamin C have lower rates of lung cancer.

Pancreatic cancer: People who eat diets rich in vitamin C and fruit have lower levels of pancreatic cancer than those who don't.

Stomach cancer: Several studies of vitamin C intake and stomach cancer establish a definitive inverse relationship. Several studies found a common bond among people who develop stomach cancer: they eat less fruits and vegetables than those who don't get cancer.

Cervical cancer: Women with low blood levels of C, or with low levels of C intake, are at greater risk of developing this form of cancer. According to a study done in Latin America in partnership with the National Cancer Institute, a high intake of vitamin C (over 314 mg per day) was associated with a 31 percent lower cervical cancer risk than in those women taking in only 153 mg of vitamin C per day. Please note that 153 mg is still more than 250 percent of the RDA.

Bladder cancer: Several studies have shown that ascorbic acid inhibits nitrosation in humans and animals and inhibits carcinogen-induced bladder tumors in animals.

Childhood brain tumors: Studies show that cancerous brain tumors are more common in children whose mother had a low level of vitamin C during pregnancy.

Breast cancer: There appears to be a strong link between low blood levels of vitamin C and breast cancer.

Colds In a study at the University of Wisconsin, Madison, Medical School, researchers exposed men who had been taking 500 mg of vitamin C, four times a day, for three and a half weeks, to cold viruses. Although the C didn't prevent colds, it did lessen the severity of symptoms such as runny noses and coughs, which is what Linus Pauling has been saying for years. Another study at Arizona State University showed that high doses of vitamin C (2000 mg daily for two weeks) can significantly lower histamine levels and may help the immune system fight against infection. However, several participants in the study developed unpleasant side effects, including diarrhea and dry nose.

Eyes Recent studies suggest that cataracts, which affect many older Americans, may be caused by cellular damage due to oxidation. Allen Taylor, director of the Laboratory for Nutrition and Vision Research at the USDA Human Nutrition Center at Tufts University, estimates that with the use of antioxidants such as vitamin C, 50 percent of all cataracts could be avoided. Tufts University researchers found that vitamin C accumulates in the eye in direct proportion to the amount consumed. When vitamin C was added to the diet of guinea pigs, their eyes showed less damage after exposure to ultraviolet light, a common cause of cataracts. Researchers also found that people given 2 grams of vitamin C a day showed less oxidative damage in their eyes. Another study, performed at Harvard Medical School, of 1380 adults showed that those who took multivitamin supplements containing antioxidants were less likely to develop cataracts than those who did not.

Heart Antioxidants, including vitamin C, are believed to help prevent blood lipids from going "rancid"; such rancidity may cause the formation of plaque in the arteries, which can lead to atherosclerosis and coronary artery disease. Studies confirm that vitamin C appears to be beneficial to the heart and circulatory system in many different ways.

At the University of California, Berkeley, researchers looked at vitamin C intakes and death rates of more than 11,000 people. They found a much lower death rate among those who took vitamin C supplements vs. those who consumed the RDA of 60 mg in their food. For men, the more vitamin C consumed, the less the risk of heart attack. Although vitamin C seemed to protect women against heart disease, the results were not as dramatic.

Another study from Berkeley showed that men who consumed low levels of vitamin C (less than 20 mg daily) had a 50 percent drop in glutathione, an amino acid and potent antioxidant that also protects against heart disease, cancer, and arthritis. When they were given vitamin C, their glutathione levels bounced back to normal. According to researchers at the USDA Human Nutrition Research Center on Aging at Tufts University, Boston, vitamin C may help prevent coronary artery disease in yet another way. Researchers studied blood vitamin C levels of men and women ranging in age from 20 to 100. Those with the highest blood levels of vitamin C had the highest levels of HDL or good cholesterol, and those with the lowest C levels had the lowest levels of good cholesterol. High vitamin C levels were also associated with lower blood pressure. High blood pressure is a major risk factor for heart attack and stroke.

High Blood Pressure Epidemiological studies have found that in populations where vitamin C intake is low, blood pressure tends to rise. David Trout, research physiologist at the Beltsville Human Nutrition Center of the U.S. Department of Agriculture, believes that people with high blood pressure need extra C. Here's why. A recent study in *Nutrition Review* found that 1000 mg of vitamin C a day significantly reduced systolic pressure (the top number) in 20 women, 12 with borderline hypertension.

Infertility Studies show that vitamin C protects human sperm from oxidative DNA damage, which may help to prevent birth defects. Bruce Ames, of the University of California at Berkeley, found that low blood levels of C are associated with genetically damaged sperm.

PERSONAL ADVICE   Vitamin C is fragile; eat fruits and vegetables raw if you can. If you want to cook them, do so for as little time as possible, with as little water as possible. Steaming is the best cooking method for retaining vitamin C. Stir-frying in a tiny amount of oil is also a good choice, because it uses as little liquid as possible and cooks the food rapidly.

Vitamin D

FACTS This fat-soluble vitamin helps the body properly utilize calcium and phosphorus to build strong teeth and bones. Vitamin D has been dubbed the "sunshine vitamin" because ultraviolet rays from the sun stimulate certain skin oils to produce vitamin D. Vitamin D is also present in a handful of foods.

Good food sources include fatty fish oils (cod, bass, mackerel, sardines, salmon, tuna, anchovies) and fortified dairy products.

Vitamin D deficiency will result in rickets, the gradual softening of bones due to poor calcification.

THE RIGHT AMOUNT The RDA for adults is 400 IU.

POSSIBLE BENEFITS

Cancer Although the exact mechanism is unknown, vitamin D is believed to help prevent colon cancer. The evidence: colon cancer rates tend to be higher in colder climates, where there is less sunlight.

Osteoporosis A USDA-sponsored study at Tufts University showed that women may be able to prevent osteoporosis by increasing vitamin D as well as calcium intake. For some time, we've known that bone loss is greater during the winter months for two reasons. First, we are less exposed to the sun, which means that our bodies are not producing as much vitamin D. Second, we get less physical exercise than in the warm months, which also reduces the amount of bone mass. The Tufts researchers wanted to see if "winter bone loss" could be treated nutritionally. In their study, 247 women were given calcium supplements bringing their total daily intake to 800 mg. Half the group received a vitamin D supplement of 400 IU, the other half received a placebo. At the end of six months, the researchers measured spine and bone density of both groups by using a highly sophisticated x-ray technique. The results: Those taking the vitamin D supplement during the winter months had only half the spinal loss of those on the calcium alone. Four 8-ounce glasses of skim milk each day would equal the amount of vitamin D consumed in study.

CAUTION Very large doses of vitamin D over a long period of time can be toxic.

Vitamin E (Tocopherol)

FACTS Vitamin E was discovered in the 1920s by two American researchers who noted that a deficiency of a particular substance isolated from food caused infertility in rats. When the substance was added back into the rats' diet, they were able to conceive. The researchers called this new vitamin tocopherol, which in Greek means to "bring forth children." Through the years, vitamin E's stock has gone up and down as researchers attempted to figure out just what exactly this vitamin does. Today, we know that vitamin E is essential for the normal functioning of the body, and is especially important for normal neurological functions in humans. Vitamin E is also a potent antioxidant, and has been dubbed the body's "first line of defense" against lipid peroxidation—that means, it protects polyunsaturated fatty acids in cell membranes from free-radical attack. Free radicals can cause the type of cellular damage that has been linked to the initiation of cancer and heart disease.

Good sources of vitamin E include vegetable oils, whole grains, peanut butter, baked sweet potato, avocado, wheat germ, almonds, peanuts, brown rice, oatmeal, mayonnaise, margarine, corn oil, peanut oil, walnuts, and other nuts.

THE RIGHT AMOUNT The RDA for vitamin E is 8 to 10 IU (with this vitamin, 1 IU is equivalent to 1 mg).

Vitamin E is synergistic with another antioxidant, selenium, which means that taking the two together greatly enhances the potency of each.

POSSIBLE BENEFITS

Antiaging Vitamin E may help protect against the ravages of aging in several ways. Studies of laboratory animals have shown that exposure to radiation appeared to rapidly age the animals and increased the level of free radicals in their cells. Adding antioxidants C and E to the diet of elderly patients in Poland decreased average blood lipid peroxide concentrations, which means it prevented harmful oxidation which can promote aging.

When patients in a nursing home in Finland were given E and selenium supplements, the staff noticed a significant improvement in their mental well-being and overall condition.

Arthritis Vitamin E appears to help alleviate the pain and stiffness of arthritis. A recent study of osteoarthritis in patients showed that vitamin E supplements helped reduce pain, improve mobility, and reduce the need for painkillers.

Cancer Vitamin E wages a three-pronged attack against cancer. First, as an antioxidant, it prevents the kind of damage to cell membranes that makes a cell ripe for cancerous changes. Second, it can aggressively fight off "bad" cells or carcinogens: it inhibits the conversion of nitrites to cancer-promoting nitrosamines in the stomach. Third, it's an immune booster, which means that it helps the immune system battle against unwanted invaders.

A major study performed at Johns Hopkins School of Hygiene and Public Health showed that low levels of vitamin E appear to increase the risk of developing lung cancer.

Heart In the 1960s, Wilfred and Evan Shute, two Canadian physicians, were ridiculed by the medical establishment for suggesting that vitamin E could prevent heart attacks. Their book, *Vitamin E for Ailing and Healthy Hearts,* was widely denounced as quackery by professionals but was popular with the public. Today, even the most conservative of cardiologists are prescribing vitamin E for a number of reasons. Several studies show that vitamin E may help improve the outcome of open heart surgery. In one study, megadoses of vitamin E were given for two weeks immediately prior to bypass surgery to 14 male patients. Another group of 14 male patients received placebos. The patients on vitamin E fared significantly better after surgery, which was reflected in improved heart function, than those who did not receive the vitamin. Researchers theorize that the vitamin E prevented the formation of free radicals, which can damage heart tissue.

Vitamin E also appears to prevent blood clots, which can result in heart attack and stroke. In one study, rats fed palm oil, high in vitamin E, showed a decrease in production of thromboxane, a potent promoter of clotting. There have been similar results in human studies. For example, estrogen, used in oral contraceptives, increases the risk of blood clots. However, this risk may be reduced by vitamin E supplementation. In one study, women taking contraceptives who were also taking vitamin E showed lower levels of clotting activity and platelet response than those observed in women not taking vitamin E. The bottom line: if you're on the pill, eat more foods rich in vitamin E or talk to your physician about taking a supplement.

Vitamin E appears to be a strong protector against heart disease for women. According to an ongoing study of more than 80,000 nurses, women in the highest 20 percent of vitamin E consumption had a 44 percent lower risk of heart disease than those in the lowest 20 percent. Women getting more than 100 mg of vitamin E had a 36 percent less risk of heart attack than those in the lowest group, who got below 30 mg of vitamin E.

But vitamin E is not for women only. A similar study of close to 40,000 male health professionals also showed that participants who consumed vitamin E supplements for two years were at a 40 percent lower risk of developing heart disease than those who did not take any supplements. In another study, researchers at the University of Texas Southwestern Medical Center in Dallas, observed 24 men ages 25 to 70, ranging from lean to obese, and from healthy to those with apparent heart conditions. One group of men received a three-month supply of soybean oil capsules; the other got identical capsules containing 900 IU of vitamin E (80 to 100 times the normal dosage). By the end of 12 weeks, the vitamin E level in the blood of those taking vitamin E was 4.4 times higher than in the other group. By the end of 6 weeks, the LDL or bad cholesterol in supplemented men sustained less than half the oxidative damage of those in the other group. Oxidative damage is believed to be responsible for the formation of plaque in the arteries.

Other studies show that people with angina, a condition characterized by pain or a tightening in the chest due to impaired blood flow, have lower than normal blood levels of vitamin E. Researchers theorize that vitamin E's anticlotting action may keep blood flowing through narrow arteries, thus preventing angina attack.

Immune Booster Studies show that vitamin E improves white blood cell activity and increases interleukin-2, a substance that promotes the production of a special kind of white cell called T cells, which help the body to fight off infection. Elderly people, who have more sluggish immune systems, should consider taking more vitamin E.

Leg Cramps Vitamin E improves the blood flow to the extremities and can help eliminate "charley horse," night cramps in the legs and hands, and other problems that often cause poor circulation.

Muscles According to a study at the Human Nutrition Research Center on Aging at Tufts, vitamin E may reduce some of the muscle damage that occurs during rigorous exercise by protecting cells from oxidation. Researchers studied 21 sedentary men, half of whom were given 800 IU of vitamin E for seven days prior to running downhill on a treadmill for 45 minutes. The other half were given placebos. After both groups exercised, the group on vitamin E excreted significantly less of a by-product of fat oxidation and had significantly lower blood levels of two substances that trigger inflammation. In other words, more gain, less pain, and less damage to body tissue. The moral of this tale: If you're planning to work out, load up on wheat germ and other vitamin-E-rich foods or take a supplement.

Ozone Protection Exposure to ultraviolet light and pollutants such as ozone and cigarette smoke can promote oxidation, which can cause cellular damage, especially to DNA. The gradual deterioration of DNA prevents the body from repairing this damage. Ozone, a major component of smog, is a very powerful oxidant that we are exposed to daily. Past studies have shown that exposure to ozone can reduce immunity to infections and, among other things, may cause damage to lung tissue and promote the growth of tumors. Lung tissue was studied in culture to determine the carcinogenic effect of ozone and the protective effect, if any, of vitamin E. The studies showed that the ozone did indeed interact with other environmental hazards to promote the growth of tumors, and that vitamin E appeared to shield the cells against these chemically induced changes. The million-dollar question is whether it will work in humans, and what level of vitamin E is needed to have a protective effect. Even without definitive answers, it's a good idea to include more vitamin-E-rich foods in your diet, especially people who live in urban areas where the exposure to pollutants is very high.

Vitamin K

FACTS A fat-soluble vitamin, K comes in two forms: vitamin K_1 is found in green, leafy vegetables; K_2 is produced in the small intestine by intestinal bacteria. Vitamin K plays many roles in the body, but its primary one is to facilitate blood clotting. Vitamin K is given to newborns to prevent bleeding because infants have underdeveloped intestinal bacteria. Recent studies suggest that vitamin K appears to help calcium absorption.

Good food sources include broccoli, alfalfa, cooked spinach, and liver.

THE RIGHT AMOUNT The RDA for adults is between 65 and 80 mcg.

People on blood thinners may develop vitamin K deficiencies.

POSSIBLE BENEFITS

Osteoporosis A recent Dutch study of postmenopausal women (ages 45 to 80) showed that calcium loss in urine could be halved by taking a daily vitamin K supplement. The inability of the body to retain calcium after menopause is believed to be a major cause of osteoporosis.

Minerals

Boron

FACTS Boron is a trace mineral that has been ignored until very recently. Boron is found in foods of plant origin, and appears to be essential for plant life. However, researchers are beginning to suspect that boron works with two other major minerals—calcium and magnesium—to promote strong bones.

Good sources of boron include nearly every type of fruit and vegetable; dried fruits, such as dried apricots and prunes, are especially rich in this mineral. Boron is not present in meat or poultry.

THE RIGHT AMOUNT To prevent osteoporosis, take 3 mg of boron daily.

POSSIBLE BENEFITS

Osteoporosis Researchers at the USDA found that a supplement of 3 mg of boron daily could double levels of serum estrogen in women, which may help prevent bone thinning caused by osteoporosis. Estrogen helps retain adequate amounts of calcium and magnesium, which are often lost during menopause, when estrogen levels dip. Calcium and magnesium help prevent the kind of bone demineralization that leads to fractures and breaks.

Calcium

FACTS Calcium is the most abundant mineral in the human body. Roughly 99 percent of the body's calcium is found in teeth and bones; 1 percent is found in fluid and soft tissues. Most people know that calcium is used to build strong bones and teeth and in maintaining bone strength, but a lesser known fact is that this mineral is also essential for the proper function of every body cell. Calcium is instrumental in muscle contraction, blood clotting, and maintenance of cell membranes. Calcium plays a critical role in the normal functioning of the heart and other muscles. Vitamin D increases calcium absorption in the body. Magnesium appears to regulate the flow of calcium between cells.

Good food sources of calcium include low-fat milk, low-fat yogurt, fortified breakfast cereals, salmon and sardines with bones, tofu (if made with calcium sulfate), and blackstrap molasses. Calcium is also present in green leafy vegetables; however, oxalic acid, found in greens such as spinach, beets, Swiss chard, and rhubarb, may hamper absorption. Protein may also hamper calcium absorption: increasing the level of protein in the body seems to increase the amount of calcium excreted in the urine. Lactose, a form of milk sugar, seems to help absorption, which is why dairy products are excellent sources of calcium.

Alcohol also impairs calcium absorption.

THE RIGHT AMOUNT The RDA for adults up to age 25 is 1200 mg, and from 25 to 50, 800 mg per day.

Some experts recommend up to 1500 mg of calcium per day for postmenopausal women who are not taking estrogen supplements. Most American women fall short of calcium. Women between the ages of 19 and 34 consume on average 665 mg per day; those between the ages of 35 and 50 take in 565 mg.

POSSIBLE BENEFITS

Cancer A recent study of men at high risk of developing colon cancer showed that increasing calcium intake lowered the rate of cell turnover in the colon dramatically; cancer is characterized by rapid cell turnover. Researchers speculate that low colon cancer rates in Finland may be due to the intake of calcium-rich dairy products. (Fiber supporters also point out that the Finns eat more fiber-rich cereals than Americans, which may also reduce their risk of colon cancer.)

Heart High cholesterol is a major risk factor for heart attack and stroke. A handful of studies suggest that calcium may be a potent "cholesterol buster." In animal studies, higher serum cholesterol levels have been observed in calcium-deficient rats. In humans, one study showed that calcium supplementation of 800 mg daily reduced blood cholesterol levels by 25 percent. Another study performed on older women showed that 750 mg supplementation of calcium reduced a mean cholesterol level of 266 mg/deciliter by 36 mg/dl. These results are promising; however, more studies are needed on calcium's role in cutting cholesterol.

High Blood Pressure Several studies have shown that calcium can lower blood pressure in animals and humans, especially for people who already have moderate to high blood pressure. James H. Dwyer of the University of Southern California School of Medicine, Los Angeles, led a study of 6634 men and women, the National Health and Nutrition Examination Survey I, which ran from 1971 to 1984. None of the participants suffered from hypertension at the beginning of the study, although many did develop it during the study. One striking finding: at any age, people who consumed at least 1 gram of calcium per day lowered their risk of developing high blood pressure by 12 percent. Some groups of people fared even better on calcium. Moderate drinkers who ate at least 1 gram of calcium per day reduced their risk of hypertension by 20 percent. (Alcohol interferes with calcium absorption.) People under the age of 40 who ate a diet of more than 1 gram of calcium per day reduced their risk of hypertension by 25 percent. Those who fared the best on calcium: slim, moderate drinkers, under 40, who ate 1 gram of calcium per day reduced their risk of hypertension by a whopping 40 percent.

Calcium also seems to help children maintain normal blood pressure. The Framingham Children's Study of 106 families tracked the dietary habits of children between the ages of 3 and 5. Based on food diaries kept by their mothers, children who ate the most calcium-rich foods had the lowest systolic blood pressure. (Systolic pressure, the top number, is generated when the heart contracts and pushes blood into the artery. Diastolic pressure, the bottom number, is the pressure in the arteries when the heart muscle relaxes between beats.)

Osteoporosis Osteoporosis, marked by a loss of bone mass and density, typically occurs in postmenopausal women and can result in breaks and fractures. Complications from osteoporosis are a leading cause of death among older women. There are several reasons osteoporosis strikes late in life. First, as we age, our bodies are not as capable of utilizing vitamin D, which makes it more difficult for the body to absorb dietary calcium. Second, the reduction of estrogen levels after menopause may also interfere with the body's ability to utilize calcium efficiently.

Although osteoporosis strikes later in life, the seeds for this debilitating and life-threatening disorder may be planted much earlier. There is some compelling evidence that a lack of calcium intake during adolescence (which is a time when many girls begin dieting) may compromise the development of peak bone mass, which could lead to osteoporosis later in life. Researchers recently examined the effect of calcium versus genetics on the bone mass development of a small group of adolescent females. The researchers expected that body build was partly inherited—girls whose mothers or fathers had big bones were expected to have bigger bones themselves. However, diet—specifically calcium intake— seemed to be an even more important factor in developing bone mass. The results of their two-year study showed that the girls taking high quantities of dietary calcium developed greater bone mass and bone density than those consuming lower levels regardless of family background. The researchers also noticed that girls taking in the highest levels of calcium (1637 mg per day) were not excreting significantly more calcium in their urine than girls on lower levels, which is a sign that the body was putting it to good use. The researchers speculate that during adolescence, when girls reach peak skeletal growth, extra calcium is retained by the body.

There is also some evidence that dietary calcium can retard bone loss in adult women. In a survey of women in twelve countries, researchers found a direct link between high calcium consumption and low risk of osteoporosis. For example, women in Finland, who consume 1300 mg of calcium daily on average, had the lowest number of fractures. Those in Japan, with the lowest consumption of calcium at 400 mg, had the highest number of fractures. However, most researchers believe that a combination of calcium and estrogen replacement is necessary to prevent osteoporosis in women who are considered at high risk of this disease.

Pregnancy Calcium may play a role in maintaining normal blood pressure during pregnancy. Studies show that in countries such as Guatemala and Ethiopia, women with diets low in calories but high in calcium have much lower levels of edema (water retention), proteinuria, and hypertension during pregnancy. A U.S. study of pregnant women confirms that calcium can help reduce high blood pressure. Researchers gave 30 women with normal blood pressure and 20 women with elevated blood pressure a 1000 mg per day calcium supplement over a 20-week period. Women with high blood pressure experienced a dramatic drop in diastolic pressure, the pressure in the arteries when the heart muscle relaxes between beats (but had no change in systolic pressure). Calcium did not appear to have any affect on women with normal blood pressure.

In yet another study of 1194 pregnant women, half received 2 grams per day of calcium, the other half a placebo. Those in the calcium group were less likely to develop hypertensive disorders such as preeclampsia, a potentially life-threatening condition that strikes roughly 7 percent of all women during the last trimester, than those in the placebo group. Although calcium won't prevent preeclampsia, it does increase the odds against it happening.

Premenstrual Syndrome Calcium-rich foods, such as warm milk, have long been a folk cure for PMS. Recently, a small study from the Human Nutrition Research Center in Grand Forks, North Dakota (*USDA Quarterly Report,* No. 2, 1991), confirms that the "old wives" may have known what they were talking about. Researchers put ten women on a high-calcium diet (1300 mg of calcium per day, half from food, half from calcium lactate supplements) and an equal number on a low-calcium diet (600 mg per day, or the average U.S. woman's daily calcium intake). Halfway through the study, the women switched protocols: the high-calcium women went on the low-calcium diet and vice versa. The overwhelming majority of women claimed that they had fewer PMS symptoms on the high-calcium diet; specifically, they were in better moods, less irritable and depressed. Several of the women on the calcium-rich diet also reported fewer headaches, backaches, and cramps. Although this was a small study, the results are promising.

Strokes Low calcium and low vitamin D intake has been linked to stroke. Researchers compared the diets of 35 women who have had strokes, with no history of high blood pressure or heart disease, with the diets of women who have never had strokes. Their findings: The healthy women's diets contained 38 percent more vitamin D and 17 percent more calcium than those of the stroke victims.

CAUTION Excessive quantities of calcium (over 2000 mg) may cause constipation and increase the risk of urinary tract infections.

Chromium

FACTS This trace mineral works with insulin in the metabolism of sugar. Chromium may help diabetics in two important ways. First, it appears to stimulate the beta cells in the pancreas to manufacture more insulin as it is needed. Second, it makes the insulin work more efficiently, thereby helping to maintain normal blood glucose levels.

Good food sources include brewer's yeast, broccoli, ham, turkey, grape juice, and shellfish.

THE RIGHT AMOUNT There is no RDA for chromium, but the average adult intake should be between 50 and 200 mcg. According to the USDA, few people get the minimum 50 mcg of this mineral. Chromium is best absorbed in the form of glucose tolerance factor (GTF), a naturally occurring compound containing chromium with niacin, glycine, glutamic acid, and cysteine. Chromium picolinate, a newer better-absorbed form of chromium, has been shown to lower cholesterol, increase life span, and may even help athletes develop muscle.

POSSIBLE BENEFITS

Heart Diabetics are at particular risk of developing coronary artery disease or having a stroke. However, a recent study suggests that chromium may reduce that risk by helping to raise HDL or "good" cholesterol. Heart patients— some with insulin-dependent diabetes and some free of diabetes—were either given a chromium supplement of 200 mcg daily for up to 16 months or given a placebo. The chromium group experienced a significant rise in HDLs as compared with the placebo group. An important finding: The diabetic patients on chromium did as well as the non-diabetic patients.

Copper

FACTS This mineral is required to convert the body's iron into hemoglobin. Copper also helps to keep bones, blood vessels, and nerves healthy and the immune system functioning normally.

Good food sources include shellfish, whole wheat, beans, nuts, seeds, prunes, calf and beef liver.

THE RIGHT AMOUNT No RDA. The National Academy of Sciences Estimated Safe and Adequate Daily Dietary Intake is 1.5 to 3 mg.

POSSIBLE BENEFITS

Arthritis Copper bracelets are a folk remedy against arthritis. Scientists used to dismiss this treatment as pure hokum; however, recently there have been some serious studies that have shown that copper bracelets do offer some relief against the pain and stiffness associated with arthritis. At one time, however, copper was considered a possible cause of arthritis. High concentrations of copper and ceruloplasmin (a protein to which copper is linked) were found in the joints of patients with rheumatoid arthritis. At first glance, it appeared as if too much copper was somehow causing this condition, but now scientists suspect that the elevated copper levels could be an attempt on the part of the body to treat itself. Studies have shown that copper included with other anti-inflammatory drugs may indeed help reduce arthritic symptoms.

Blood Clots Could heart disease be caused by inadequate copper intake? Researchers have found many similarities between copper-deficient animals and human heart disease patients. According to a recent USDA study, copper-deficient mice took 2.5 times longer to dissolve blood clots than mice taking in the proper amount of this mineral. Similar tests performed on humans also show that heart patients take longer to dissolve clots, which may explain the cause of their heart disease. Tiny blood clots can join with cholesterol and other debris to form plaque, which clogs arteries, eventually impairing the flow of blood to the heart and other organs. If the artery becomes too narrow, it can result in a heart attack. A piece of plaque breaking off and entering the bloodstream can also cause a heart attack or stroke.

Fluoride

FACTS This mineral is essential in the formation of teeth and bone.

Fluoride is available in seafood, in gelatin, and in the drinking water in about 45 percent of all communities in the United States.

THE RIGHT AMOUNT No RDA. The National Academy of Sciences Estimated Safe and Adequate Dietary Intake is between 1.5 and 4 mg. If your water supply is fluoridated, you probably don't require any additional fluoride. If it isn't, talk to your dentist or physician about taking a supplement. Doses exceeding 20 mg per day can produce toxic effects.

POSSIBLE BENEFITS

Cavities In the 1930s, researchers noticed that there was an inverse relationship between fluoride levels in the drinking water and the prevalence of tooth decay. In the 1950s, many communities across the United States began to fluoridate their drinking water, and the results have been dramatic. In some communities, children who drink fluoridated water have up to 60 percent fewer cavities than those who do not. In communities where fluoride levels are low, dentists often give patients extra fluoride treatments.

Osteoporosis Several studies suggest that people who live in areas with optimal levels of fluoride in the water supply are at lower risk of developing osteoporosis and other skeletal problems, including reduced bone density and collapsed vertebrae.

Iodine

FACTS Iodine is a micronutrient that is instrumental in the functioning of the thyroid gland, which produces the hormones that regulate many body functions.

Iodine deficiency can result in hypothyroidism (an underactive thyroid), which is characterized by extreme lethargy, puffiness under the chin, weight gain, and feeling cold.

Good food sources include seafood, seaweed, iodized salt, and kelp.

THE RIGHT AMOUNT The RDA is 150 mcg for adults.

Pregnant women need 175 mcg; lactating women require 200 mcg.

Iron

FACTS Iron is necessary for the production of hemoglobin, red blood cell corpuscles, and myoglobin, the red pigment in muscles and certain enzymes. Heme iron, found in animal products, is easier to absorb than iron found in plants. Vitamin C helps facilitate absorption of iron, while calcium and caffeine may hamper absorption. Women who menstruate need extra iron to compensate for their monthly blood loss. An iron-poor diet is linked to learning problems in children and to difficulty concentrating and a short attention span in young women. Iron deficiency can lead to iron-deficiency anemia, characterized by fatigue, feeling cold, and lowered immunity.

Too much iron can be as harmful as too little. High levels of iron stored in the body can contribute to the risk of developing coronary artery disease. One Finnish study focused on 1931 men who, at start of study in 1984, had no sign of heart disease. Researchers found that men who had diets higher in iron-rich foods were more likely to develop heart disease. In addition, those with high concentrations of iron in their blood, more than 200 micrograms per liter, were twice as likely to suffer from heart attack as those with lower ferritin levels. Scientists hypothesize that too much iron in the blood can promote formation of free radicals, which can injure the cells lining the artery walls and damage heart muscles. (A good antioxidant supplement would prevent this problem.)

Good food sources include pork, oysters, clams, beef, liver, chicken, and turkey. Dried fruit, green vegetables, and beans are also reasonably good sources, although not as good as meat.

THE RIGHT AMOUNT The RDA is 15 mg for women age 11 to 50. It drops to 10 mg for women over 50. (Menopause is the dividing line.)

Pregnant women need 30 mg daily.

The RDA for men is 10 mg.

About 75 percent of all American women 19 to 50 have iron intakes below 80 percent of RDA.

POSSIBLE BENEFITS

Iron-Deficiency Anemia Perhaps as many as 15 percent of all menstruating women have an iron deficiency. Anemia, a condition that impairs the body's ability to produce healthy red blood cells, occurs if blood iron levels fall below 12 mcg per liter of blood and hemoglobin levels fall below 12.5 grams per 100 ml of blood. People who are anemic tend to tire easily, and are more susceptible to infection. Women are especially prone to anemia because they menstruate and are more likely to be on a diet than are men. Vegetarians who do not eat meat are also at risk of developing anemia and must be especially careful to eat dried fruits, beans, and iron-fortified grains.

CAUTION If you suspect that you are iron-deficient, consult with your physician before taking any iron supplements. Excess iron can be toxic, if not taken with the appropriate antioxidants.

Magnesium

FACTS This mineral is used for a wide variety of body functions, including building bones, manufacturing proteins, releasing energy from muscle storage, and regulating body temperature. Magnesium is necessary for vitamin C and calcium metabolism, as well as that of phosphorus, sodium, and potassium. Magnesium works against calcium in regulating heartbeat and muscle contraction: magnesium relaxes blood vessels; calcium causes them to constrict. Too little magnesium allows for the buildup of calcium and sodium (two constricting agents) in the body, which can interfere with the blood flow into small arteries, thus causing high blood pressure. A normal mineral balance is essential for normal heart and cell function.

Low intake is associated with high blood pressure, heart arrhythmias, and heart attack.

Good food sources include wheat bran, whole grains, leafy green vegetables, milk, meat, beans, bananas, apricots, dry mustard, curry powder, and cocoa.

THE RIGHT AMOUNT The RDA for adults is 250 to 350 mg daily.

Pregnant and lactating women need 300 to 355 mg per day.

POSSIBLE BENEFITS

Diabetes and High Blood Pressure More than 80 percent of people with diabetes die of some form of cardiovascular disease. High blood pressure, a major complication of diabetes, dramatically increases the risk of heart attack or stroke. Magnesium may help noninsulin-dependent diabetics maintain normal blood pressure. Noninsulin-dependent diabetes mellitus is characterized by elevated levels of insulin and glucose in the blood. (Glucose is a sugar that cells break down to produce energy.) Unlike insulin-dependent diabetes, in which the body is unable to make insulin, in this form of the disease, insulin-resistant diabetes, the body produces insulin but cannot use it efficiently to turn glucose into energy. A recent study (reported at the American Heart Association's 1990 meeting on high blood pressure) established a link between high calcium levels and low magnesium levels in people with this form of diabetes and high blood pressure. In a second study performed at the City of Hope Medical Center in Duarte, California, magnesium supplements of 400 mg per day dramatically lowered blood pressure in people with this type of diabetes. Although more research needs to be done, insulin-resistant diabetics should make sure that they are eating a magnesium-rich diet. In addition, they should talk to their physicians about taking a magnesium supplement.

Glucose Handling Older people can become insulin-resistant, that is, they cannot use insulin efficiently to turn glucose into energy, thus glucose levels rise. Insulin resistance increases the risk of developing diabetes and high blood pressure. According to an article in the *American Journal of Clinical Nutrition*, older people can improve their ability to metabolize glucose by taking magnesium supplements.

Heart Magnesium may be just what the physician orders after a heart attack. In a study sponsored by the National Heart, Lung and Blood Institute in Bethesda, Maryland, magnesium was given intravenously to a group of heart patients immediately following a heart attack. The findings: Those given magnesium had a 55 percent higher survival rate than those who had not been given this mineral.

Other studies show that magnesium may protect against the formation of dangerous blood clots by preventing platelets (part of the blood) from clumping together. Blood clots can cause heart attack and stroke.

Migraine Women who have migraines tend to get headaches during or right before their periods. A recent article in *Headache* reports that women who take 200 mg of magnesium daily have significantly fewer headaches in general, especially during their periods.

Premature Labor Some obstetricians recommend that their patients take a magnesium supplement during pregnancy to prevent premature labor. In fact, high doses of magnesium are given intravenously to prevent preterm labor in women who are showing signs of contractions. Magnesium helps to relax the muscles of the uterus, working against calcium, which facilitates the chemical reaction that is responsible for labor. Pregnant women should be especially vigilant about eating enough magnesium-rich foods. (Check with your obstetrician before taking this or any other drug or supplement during pregnancy.)

Premenstrual Syndrome Research has shown that women with PMS have low blood levels of magnesium. In a recent study published in *Obstetrics and Gynecology*, women who suffered from PMS were given either 350 mg of magnesium or a placebo three times daily during the last two weeks of the menstrual cycle. The PMS symptoms, including moodiness, bloating, aches and pains, were significantly reduced among the magnesium takers.

CAUTION Excess magnesium can cause diarrhea and throw off your mineral balance. Do not exceed doses of 1000 mg per day.

Manganese

FACTS Although we need only a tiny amount of this trace element, it appears to have many essential jobs in the body. Manganese helps activate the enzymes that are necessary for the proper use of vitamin C, biotin, and B_1 (thiamine). It is an important player in the metabolism of food and in the production of fatty acids and cholesterol. It is also important for the normal functioning of the nervous system and for the production of sex hormones. Manganese is an antioxidant, and as such may play a role in preventing cancer and heart disease. However, there hasn't been a lot of research devoted to manganese, but that may change.

Good food sources are nuts, whole grains, green leafy vegetables, peas, beets, and egg yolks.

THE RIGHT AMOUNT No RDA, but 2.5 to 5 mg is considered the daily requirement for adults.

Phosphorus

FACTS This mineral is abundant in the American diet and is present in virtually every cell. Phosphorus helps to build strong teeth and bones, and is also instrumental in the release of energy from our food and in the formation of genetic material, cell membranes, and many enzymes. Calcium and phosphorus should be at a 2:1 balance to work correctly. Phosphorus deficiencies are rare.

THE RIGHT AMOUNT The RDA is 1200 mg for teenagers and young adults (11 to 24).

The RDA for adults over 25 is 800 mg.

POSSIBLE BENEFITS Although your body could not function without phosphorus, it is not as of yet used to treat or
prevent particular ailments.

Potassium

FACTS This mineral works with sodium to regulate the
body's water balance and normalize heart rhythm. It is also
critical for the normal functioning of nerves and muscles.
Low intake is associated with high blood pressure and heart
arrhythmias.

Good food sources include white potato (at 500 mg one
of the best), winter squash, dried apricots, plain low-fat
yogurt, banana, lima beans, orange juice, prunes, and baked
sweet potato.

THE RIGHT AMOUNT No RDA. The National Academy of
Sciences proposed range of Estimated Safe and Adequate
Daily Dietary Intake for potassium is 1600 to 2000 mg
minimum. I recommend at least 2000 mg daily.

POSSIBLE BENEFITS

High Blood Pressure Increasing dietary potassium may
reduce the need for antihypertensive medication in some
patients. In a recent study of 54 patients with high blood
pressure, half were given information on increasing their
dietary intake of potassium; the other half stuck with their
regular diets. Researchers monitored the potassium intake
of both groups of patients each month. Those taking the
added potassium were able to significantly reduce their need
for blood pressure medication. By the end of the study, 81

percent of patients on potassium-rich diets could control their blood pressure by using less than 50 percent of the initial therapy. An added bonus: Patients in the high-potassium group felt better and had fewer symptoms. In summarizing their conclusions to the study, published in the *Annals of Internal Medicine,* researchers noted, "Increasing the dietary potassium intake from natural foods is a feasible and effective measure to reduce antihypertensive treatment."

CAUTION Excess potassium is normally excreted by the kidney. However, people with kidney failure should not eat foods high in potassium or take potassium supplements.

Selenium

FACTS Although you only need a tiny amount of this essential trace mineral, it is of critical importance. Working together with glutathione, a tripeptide found in the body, selenium is a major antioxidant serving as a free-radical scavenger. It also detoxifies toxic metals such as mercury, cadmium, and arsenic as well as other potentially carcinogenic substances, by binding with them to form compounds that are flushed out of the system. Studies suggest that selenium may detoxify peroxidized fats, which, if left to their own devices, may contribute to the growth of cancerous tumors.

Good food sources include garlic, onions, fish, shellfish, red meat, red grapes, broccoli, whole wheat and grains (processing wheat to white flour reduces selenium content by 75 percent!), eggs, organ meats, and chicken. The amount of selenium in vegetables varies depending on the soil content.

THE RIGHT AMOUNT For nearly two decades I have been singing the praises of this mineral. Finally, in 1990, the U.S. government acknowledged its importance by setting an RDA of 50 to 100 mcg daily. I think that may be low: cancer researchers contend that at least 200 mcg a day is needed to protect against cancer.

CAUTION Doses of over 200 mcg may be toxic.

POSSIBLE BENEFITS

Cancer There is convincing evidence that selenium may help protect against cancer. Selenium levels in soil vary from country to country and, in the United States, from state to state: studies show that the states with the highest levels of selenium have the lowest rates of cancer. Other studies show that populations with the highest blood selenium levels have the lowest cancer rates. Mice fed a high diet in polyunsaturated fats and low in selenium developed breast tumors; those fed polyunsaturated fats and selenium did not.

Heart Selenium—perhaps due to its antioxidant activity—also appears to protect against heart and circulatory diseases. The states with the lowest selenium levels in their soil have the highest rate of stroke in the United States— the so-called southwestern Stroke Belt.

Sodium

FACTS Sodium is an important element in blood that, along with potassium, helps the body to maintain a normal fluid balance. We get sodium from our diet in the form of sodium chloride or table salt. Although sodium is essential for life, too much sodium can cause problems. People who eat a highly salty diet are at greater risk of developing stomach and other forms of gastrointestinal cancers. In addition, salt may cause high blood pressure in many people. In order to maintain a normal salt and water balance in the body, excess salt is excreted in urine. However, some people may have a condition known as salt sensitivity, in which they retain excess salt. In order to compensate for this sodium overload, their body tissues hold on to excess water. As a result, their blood volume increases, their heart must work all the harder to pump the excess fluid, and their blood pressure rises. How can you tell if you are "salt sensitive"? If you have high blood pressure, you can try reducing your salt intake and see if it makes a difference. If your pressure begins going down, chances are you've been eating too much salt.

THE RIGHT AMOUNT   Most Americans consume at least two to three times the amount of salt that they actually should. The American Heart Association recommends limiting your salt intake to 2400 mg per day, or to 1000 mg per 1000 calories. In order to comply with these guidelines, you may have to adjust your eating habits. One meal in a fastfood restaurant could easily eat up those 2000 mg. (Just the hamburger alone weighs in at 1200 mg of sodium.) If you're not careful, a dinner in a Japanese restaurant could do the same: just a single tablespoon of soy sauce has about 800 mg. (If you use soy sauce, buy the salt-reduced variety.) Watch the salt shaker! It's easy to go overboard.

Zinc

FACTS This mineral plays an important role in cell division, growth, and repair. Because of its role in cell division, it is also very important for wound healing, which requires the rapid production of new cells. Zinc is instrumental in maintaining a normal sense of taste and smell and appears to be an immune booster.

Zinc is also critical for the proper functioning of the male reproductive system.

Good food sources include lamb chops, oysters, pork, liver, eggs, brewer's yeast, milk, beans, wheat germ, pumpkin seeds.

THE RIGHT AMOUNT The RDA for women is 12 mg. Pregnant women need 15 mg daily. The RDA for men is 15 mg.

POSSIBLE BENEFITS

Colds Zinc may be the most effective treatment against one of humankind's most annoying problems—the common cold. Recently, 73 Dartmouth College students with colds were given a new form of zinc lozenges at the earliest stages of their illness. The dose: two lozenges every two hours, up to eight per day. The results: The lozenges reduced the duration of the cold by more than 40 percent (from the average nine days to five days) and also greatly reduced the severity of cold symptoms. Based on this study, conducted by the husband and wife team, John C. Godfrey, Ph.D., and Nancy Godfrey, Ph.D., zinc works even better than vitamin C in taming a cold. Although zinc lozenges are widely available in natural food stores and pharmacies, the couple claim that they have developed a more potent version which is not yet available in the United States.

Male Infertility There are heavy concentrations of zinc in the male prostate gland, which manufactures prostatic fluid, in which sperm cells are mixed to make semen. Mild zinc deficiency can lead to a low sperm count, a major cause of male infertility. Zinc is also believed to regulate the metabolism of testosterone in the prostate, the male hormone that regulates sex drive. (Interesting enough, oysters, which are very rich in zinc, are often touted as a male aphrodisiac.) I have heard of several cases in which male infertility was overcome by the addition of a zinc supplement in the diet.

Zinc may also help to prevent enlargement of the prostate gland, which is a frequent problem among older men.

CHAPTER 4

The "Hot Hundred": From Alfalfa to Yogurt

Every day we make important choices about our health. What we choose to eat is perhaps one of the most important of those choices. However, many of us do not choose wisely. Some people may be genuinely confused about which foods are better than others. Some are simply too busy to ponder everything they eat. This chapter, however, will make it a lot easier for you to eat both wisely and well. Out of the thousands of different foods that are available, I have compiled a list of the "Hot Hundred" foods, which I feel offer the greatest health potential at this time.

I have selected a wide range of foods because I feel that a well-balanced diet is the best way to prevent nutritional deficiencies.

Many of the foods in the "Hot Hundred" have earned their place among this group because of their healing ingredients: some are rich in phytochemicals; some are packed with fiber; some are terrific sources of particular vitamins or minerals that may protect against various ailments. However, some foods in the "Hot Hundred" have been selected because of the things that they lack—notably fat (a major culprit for many different diseases) and/or toxins which can be potentially dangerous.

Most important, all of the foods listed in the "Hot Hundred" met another important criteria—they taste good. I know that it's impossible to stick to a healthy eating plan if you can't stomach the food!

After reading this chapter, you will see that it is easier than you think to take advantage of nature's healing foods.

Alfalfa

FACTS Dubbed the "great healer" by noted biologist Frank Bouer, alfalfa sprouts are low in things that you don't want—calories and fat—but are high in fiber. Bouer discovered that the leaves of the alfalfa plant contain eight essential enzymes. Alfalfa has been used in herbal medicine for years, but its potential healing properties are just beginning to be recognized by modern science.

Alfalfa may also be a potent natural cholesterol buster, according to a recent study that appeared in the scientific journal *Atherosclerosis*. Researchers gave 15 patients with high cholesterol 40 grams of alfalfa seeds three times daily for eight weeks. The result: the median total cholesterol declined by 17 percent, and better yet, the LDL or "bad" cholesterol dropped by 18 percent. This study confirms the results of several others that show that alfalfa can be an effective treatment in combatting high cholesterol.

Alfalfa is also a good source of vitamin K, which facilitates blood clotting and helps to prevent hemorrhaging. Vitamin K also appears to help the body retain calcium.

POSSIBLE BENEFITS By cutting cholesterol and reducing harmful LDLs, alfalfa may help to prevent coronary artery disease and stroke.

Vitamin K may help prevent osteoporosis by preventing the loss of calcium in the urine.

CAUTION People with lupus or other autoimmune diseases should steer clear of alfalfa. Several studies show that L-canavanine, a compound found in alfalfa, can trigger an autoimmune response in the body similar to lupus.

PERSONAL ADVICE Alfalfa sprouts make a good-tasting and healthy garnish on a sandwich or a mixed salad.

Almonds

FACTS It may sound pretty nutty, but even though almonds are very high in fat (13 grams per ounce) they may be good for your heart! A major study of 26,000 members of the Seventh-Day Adventist Church showed that those who ate almonds, peanuts, and walnuts at least six times a week had an average life span of seven years longer than the general population, and a substantially lower rate of heart attack. Almonds are rich in monounsaturated fatty acids, which reduce cholesterol, and thus may protect against heart disease. Almonds are also high in vitamin E, another heart "protector."

Almonds have an edge over other nuts because they are also an excellent nondairy source of calcium: one ounce of almonds provides around 10 percent of the RDA for this mineral.

POSSIBLE BENEFITS Monounsaturated fatty acids help keep cholesterol in check.

Vitamin E, a potent antioxidant, helps to prevent the accumulation of plaque in the arteries, which can lead to a heart attack.

Calcium helps build strong bones and also helps regulate heartbeat and normalize blood pressure.

Amaranth

FACTS Amaranth, a grain that was highly prized by the Aztecs more than 500 years ago, is being rediscovered by health-conscious Americans today. A small seed that resembles millet (and has a mild, nutty flavor), amaranth cooks up into a very tasty cereal or main dish. It can also be toasted and used to spice up soups, salads or stew. Amaranth is rich in lysine, one of the eight essential amino acids that the body cannot produce itself, and is usually missing in plant food (but is abundant in animal protein). Amaranth is also very high in iron and calcium, two minerals that are often lacking from the diets of women and girls. A 2-ounce serving of cooked amaranth contains 80 percent of the RDA for iron and 10 percent of the RDA for calcium. Amaranth is also low in fat and calories and high in fiber.

POSSIBLE BENEFITS Amaranth offers high-quality protein without the added fat or calories of meat.

Iron is necessary for the formation of red blood cells. Women who menstruate often do not get enough iron and can end up anemic.

Calcium is essential for strong teeth and bones, as well as normal blood pressure. Girls and women in particular need calcium to prevent osteoporosis, or thinning of the bones, in later life. Calcium may also help to prevent various kinds of cancer.

Fiber helps to maintain bowel regularity and prevent colon and rectal cancer.

PERSONAL ADVICE There are several amaranth products, from amaranth flakes to amaranth cookies and granola, being sold on the market. Many of these products contain very little amaranth, and thus offer little advantage over other grain products. To avoid being short-changed, buy real amaranth seed and cook it yourself. I like it seasoned with a little soy sauce; however, some people prefer to sweeten it with brown sugar.

Anchovy

FACTS Some people eat them on pizza, others toss them in a salad, and still others throw them in the blender with some oil, vinegar, and spices to make a tangy salad dressing. However you eat them, anchovies are packed with good things. A 3½-ounce serving has 127 calories and 4.8 grams of fat, including an impressive 1.4 grams of omega-3 fatty acids. According to the National Heart and Lung Institute, eating even 1 gram of omega-3 fatty acids daily can reduce a man's risk of developing coronary artery disease by 40 percent. (The studies were performed on men.) Omega-3 fatty acids can also be of great benefit to women: they reduce blood triglyceride levels; levels over 190 mg/dl substantially increase the risk of heart attack in women. (Levels over 400 mg/dl increase the risk of heart disease in men.)

Anchovies are also rich in nucleic acids, RNA and DNA,

substances that some researchers believe may retard the aging process. The body is made up of millions of cells, the average cell having a life span of roughly two years. Before a cell dies, it reproduces itself, but with each reproduction, it goes through some changes, not necessarily for the better. In other words, it begins to wear out. Nucleic acids may help produce healthier cells that are able to live longer, retarding the aging process.

Anchovies also have a fair amount of vitamin A and calcium; both are known protectors against heart disease and cancer.

POSSIBLE BENEFITS Omega-3 fatty acids:

♦ Can cut cholesterol and triglycerides, thus reducing the risk of developing coronary artery disease
♦ Reduce the risk of blood clots and lower blood pressure, two risk factors associated with stroke and heart attack
♦ Modulate prostaglandin metabolism—excess production of certain prostaglandins is linked to tumor production in animals, and is believed to play a role in inflammatory diseases such as arthritis and psoriasis
♦ Are present in breast milk, and are essential for normal brain and eye development

Nucleic acids may prevent premature aging.

PERSONAL ADVICE To reduce salt content, soak anchovies in a bowl of cold milk or water in the refrigerator for several hours.

Apple

FACTS An apple a day may keep the cardiologist away. Apple is rich in pectin, a form of soluble fiber that has been shown to reduce cholesterol. In fact, one medium-size, unpeeled apple provides 3.5 grams of fiber—more than 10 percent of the daily fiber intake recommended by nutrition experts—at a relatively spare 80 calories. (Without the peel, an apple provides a very respectable 2.7 grams of fiber.)

The pectin in apple not only reduces cholesterol but appears to target the "bad" cholesterol. This was tested in a study of two strains of hamsters. One group of hamsters with normal cholesterol levels was fed apples in addition to their regular diet. Another group of hamsters, specifically bred to develop high cholesterol, was also fed a normal diet in addition to apples. According to this study, both groups of hamsters benefitted by eating apples, but in different ways. The normal-cholesterol group showed a 20 percent drop in their cholesterol levels. The addition of apples to the diet of the high-cholesterol group appeared to normalize their cholesterol. Even better, those eating apples showed a decrease in LDL or "bad" cholesterol, the kind that clogs arteries and blocks blood from reaching vital organs such as the brain and the heart. The same researchers performed several similar studies on human subjects and discovered that by eating two apples a day, people can also reduce their cholesterol by as much as 16 percent.

An added bonus: Apples are also good for diabetics, because soluble fiber helps regulate blood sugar, preventing a sudden increase or drop in serum sugar levels.

POSSIBLE BENEFITS Helps prevent heart disease by reducing cholesterol levels.

Helps maintain normal blood sugar.

PERSONAL ADVICE Apples are one of several fruits that are not only treated with insecticides but also sprayed with a coating of wax to prevent moisture loss and give a shiny appearance. Scrubbing the apple well in cool water before eating it will help remove some but not all of the wax and insecticides. I don't advise peeling the apple, because you lose much of the valuable pectin in the skin. Therefore, your best bet is to buy apples from a supermarket that can certify, based on its own laboratory tests, that the produce it sells has minimal levels of insecticides and other potentially harmful chemicals. However, if you're skittish about consuming any chemicals that you don't need, buy organic apples, which may cost a bit more, but offer greater peace of mind.

Apricot

FACTS Why are apricots so good for you? The answer: beta-carotene. Fresh or dried, apricots are abundant in this plant form of vitamin A. Three small fresh apricots (considered to be one serving by the USDA) have 2770 IU of beta-carotene, or more than 50 percent of the RDA—all for about 50 calories.

Although dried apricots are higher in calories, they have a nutritional edge over fresh. One-half cup of dried apricots (165 calories) has nearly a whole day's supply of beta-carotene, as well as a hefty serving of potassium and boron, and roughly 20 percent of the RDA for iron (which is quite impressive for a nonmeat source). Dried apricots are also higher in fiber than fresh and, like fresh, have virtually no sodium or fat.

POSSIBLE BENEFITS People who eat foods rich in beta-carotene have lower levels of cancer than people who don't.

A potent antioxidant, beta-carotene may prevent the formation of plaque deposits in arteries, which can lead to coronary artery disease.

Potassium helps to maintain the normal fluid balance in the body and helps to normalize blood pressure and heart function.

Boron may help to prevent osteoporosis by helping postmenopausal women retain estrogen, which facilitates calcium absorption.

Iron is essential for the formation of red blood cells. An iron deficiency can cause fatigue and weaken resistance against infection.

CAUTION Sulfites are often added to fruit during the drying process to maintain color and to preserve beta-carotene. Although most people can tolerate sulfites with no problem, about 1 million Americans, mostly asthmatics, are allergic to this preservative and can have a severe reaction to it. If you are asthmatic or highly allergic and want to eat dried fruit, read the label carefully. The FDA requires that food manufacturers list sulfites clearly on the package. Sulfite-free fruit is available at natural food stores.

Asparagus

FACTS For thousands of years, Chinese herbalists have used asparagus root to treat a wide range of ills, from arthritis to infertility. Asparagus root contains compounds called steroidal glycosides, which may have anti-inflammatory properties. Although Western medicine doesn't recognize asparagus as a cure, it is beginning to acknowledge that foods like asparagus contain lots of vitamins and minerals that can help keep you healthy.

Just ½ cup of cooked asparagus can provide roughly 100 mcg of folic acid (about 25 percent of the RDA) and 49 mg of vitamin C (a hefty amount, considering the RDA for nonsmokers is 60 mg). Asparagus is also a fair source of potassium and beta-carotene.

Asparagus is a natural diuretic.

Few serious scientific studies have been done on asparagus, which is surprising considering its long history as an herbal medicine. However, in 1991, one Italian researcher reported that a compound in asparagus had shown some antiviral activity in test tube studies. Hopefully, this result will pique the interest of other researchers.

POSSIBLE BENEFITS Folic acid may help to prevent birth defects, cervical cancer, colon and rectal cancer, and heart disease.

Vitamin C may protect against cancer and heart disease and also helps boost the immune system.

Beta-carotene may help protect against cancer and heart disease.

Potassium helps regulate the electrolyte balance within each cell, and also helps to maintain normal heart function and blood pressure.

Asparagus can help prevent water retention.

Banana

FACTS This yellow-skin fruit proves the adage that good things really do come in small packages. The average banana contains 451 mg of potassium, a mineral that is essential for normal blood pressure and heart function. In a recent study of patients being treated for high blood pressure, those who were put on a diet high in potassium were able to significantly reduce or eliminate their medication.

Banana also has more than 25 percent of the RDA for vitamin B_6, and about 15 percent of the RDA for vitamin C (for nonsmokers).

At 105 calories and virtually no fat, a banana is a great between-meal snack.

POSSIBLE BENEFITS Potassium helps to maintain normal fluid and electrolyte balance in the body's cells.

By regulating blood pressure and heart function, the potassium in banana helps prevent heart attack, stroke, and dangerous heart arrhythmias.

Vitamin B_6 is a natural immune booster. Combined with vitamin C, it helps your body fight infection.

PERSONAL ADVICE A little-known fact about bananas—this fruit is also a natural antacid. If you suffer from heartburn, try eating a banana to quell the fires inside. I've done it and it works!

Anyone who is taking a diuretic for high blood pressure should eat a banana or two a day to replenish the lost potassium that is literally washed out of the body. (Never use a diuretic unless you are under a physician's supervision—these drugs can have serious side effects.)

Banana is possibly the world's most perfect food. I've often said, if I was stranded on a desert island, the two things I would need to survive would be a banana tree and water.

Barley

FACTS I'm willing to wager that many members of the "fast-food" generation may never even have tasted this wonderful grain. However, as they mature and become more concerned about preventing a heart attack than succumbing to a "Big Mac" Attack, they may actually begin to seek this grain out.

Barley, an excellent source of soluble fiber, has been shown to lower blood cholesterol levels. A recent Australian study of 21 men with mildly high cholesterol levels showed that when they were given a diet rich in barley products, their cholesterol levels dropped an average of 6 percent overall. More good news—the LDL or "bad" cholesterol declined by 7 percent. A similar test performed at Montana State University yielded even better results: people given a high barley diet showed a 12 percent drop in cholesterol.

POSSIBLE BENEFITS Helps prevent coronary artery disease and stroke by cutting overall cholesterol and LDLs.

PERSONAL ADVICE There are some new quick-cooking barley products on the market that take about ten minutes to prepare. Try them for breakfast. Season with a dab of low-fat margarine or a touch of maple syrup and a sprinkle of cinnamon.

Bass (Sea)

FACTS A friend of mine was distraught over a recent story in a leading consumer magazine describing how dangerous toxins in our waters were winding up in fish. "I've given up steak, I've stopped going to McDonald's, pizza's too high in fat, and hot dogs are full of nitrites. Do I have to give up fish, too?" Much to his relief, I told him that in most cases fish was still "safe," especially if he spread the risk by eating a wide variety of fish raised in different waters. That way, he wouldn't be consuming too much of any particular toxin. However, some fish are safer than others, and because it is caught offshore where the waters are less polluted, sea bass is one of the safest. (Don't confuse sea bass with striped bass, which can be tainted with toxic PCBs.)

Sea bass is also one of the healthiest fish. It is low in saturated fat, low in calories, and has a half a gram of omega-3 fatty acids in every 4-ounce serving. Even though it is not as rich in omega-3 as some other fish, even a small amount of fish oil goes a long way. According to the National Heart and Lung Institute, just 1.0 gram of omega-3 fatty acid daily may reduce the risk of cardiovascular disease in men by 40 percent. In addition, since toxins are stored in fatty tissue, it stands to reason that a low-fat fish will be less toxic.

POSSIBLE BENEFITS A low-fat diet protects against heart disease, stroke and certain forms of cancer.

Omega-3 fatty acids:

♦ Lower cholesterol and triglycerides, reducing the risk of developing coronary artery disease

♦ Can lower blood pressure and prevent dangerous blood clots, thus protecting against both heart attack and stroke
♦ May inhibit the growth of cancerous tumors
♦ Have anti-inflammatory properties, and may be useful in the treatment of arthritis, psoriasis, lupus, asthma, and ulcerative colitis
♦ Are present in breast milk and essential for normal brain and eye development

Beansprouts (Mung Bean)

FACTS They're extremely low-calorie and high in vitamin C—1 cup provides half the RDA for nonsmokers. Add to this 1.6 grams of fiber per cup and you've got a food worthy of inclusion into any diet. Beansprouts are the mainstay of Oriental cuisines, but that doesn't mean that they don't mix well with American fare. Try throwing them into your salad, using them instead of lettuce on a sandwich, or eating them alone.

POSSIBLE BENEFITS Vitamin C helps protect against cancer and heart disease. It also helps the body fight against infection.

Fiber helps to maintain bowel regularity and protects against colon and rectal cancers.

Beef Tenderloin

FACTS Many fat and cholesterol watchers may think that they can never indulge in a piece of meat, but they are wrong. Although some cuts of meat are both fattening and fatty, beef tenderloin (which is cut into filet mignon) is an excellent food choice, for many reasons. First, it is relatively low in fat and calories: a 3-ounce serving of lean tenderloin is 170 calories and 8 grams of fat. Beef is also packed with important vitamins and minerals. Lean beef is a good source of B vitamins such as B_{12}, riboflavin, B_6, and niacin. A 3-ounce portion (about the size of a deck of cards) provides about 20 percent of the RDA for iron, a fair amount of potassium, and nearly 40 percent of the RDA for zinc. In fact, ounce for ounce, lean beef is one of the most nutrient-rich foods around.

POSSIBLE BENEFITS Iron and vitamin B_{12} can help prevent anemia. The kind of heme iron found in beef is more easily absorbed by the body than iron found in vegetable or grain sources.

B_{12} deficiency in older adults can cause memory loss, confusion, mood changes—all neurological changes that can easily be mistaken for senility.

Zinc and vitamin B_6 are important immune boosters.

B vitamins in general are important for the conversion of food to energy.

PERSONAL ADVICE A little beef goes a long way . . . watch your portion size!

Black Beans

FACTS We in the West used to take pity on the less affluent people of the world who were forced to subsist on rice and beans, while we gorged on meat and potatoes. In the early

1970s, researcher Denis Burkitt set us straight. Dr. Burkitt and his colleagues published a paper that linked colon cancer—which is common in the United States but rare in Africa and other Third World areas—to the lack of fiber in our diets. Dr. Burkitt theorized that fiber speeds up the time food spends in the colon. As food is digested, potential carcinogens—some occur naturally in food, others are from insecticides or processing—become more concentrated; thus the faster food is passed through the body, the less exposure to cancer-causing chemicals. A high-fat diet is also believed to promote various forms of cancer because carcinogenic toxins are stored in fatty tissue in the body.

Black beans can help prevent cancer because they are high in fiber and low in fat and calories. A ½ cup serving contains more than 6 grams of dietary fiber along with a fair amount of potassium, zinc, iron, and B vitamins. Like meat, black beans are a good source of protein, although they lack lysine and other essential amino acids that make a protein complete. However, the addition of a grain such as corn or rice can turn a plate of black beans into a well-balanced meal.

POSSIBLE BENEFITS   Several studies have shown that the fiber in beans can help lower blood cholesterol levels, which in turn can reduce the risk of diabetes, heart attack, and stroke.

A high-fiber diet appears to protect against colon/rectal cancer.

Blackstrap Molasses

FACTS   Back in the old days—long before the typical American breakfast consisted of bleached-out white bread doused with fat—our forefathers were eating slices of crusty whole grain bread slathered with blackstrap molasses.

Thick and sweet, blackstrap molasses is packed with good things. Two tablespoons contain 274 mg of calcium (nearly as much as a glass of milk), which makes it one of the best nondairy sources of this mineral. It is also loaded with two other vital minerals—potassium (1171 mg) and iron (at 10 mg, close to 40 percent of the RDA for women). It is not low-calorie, weighing in at 85 calories, but these are far from "empty calories."

There are three different kinds of molasses: unsulfured, sulfured, and blackstrap. Blackstrap molasses, the most concentrated and carmelized type, is the syrup that remains after the sugar cane is made into table sugar. The lighter molasses has only a fraction of the nutrients of blackstrap molasses.

Although you may not want to pour blackstrap molasses on your bread, it can be used in baking as a healthier alternative to sugar. In fact, during Colonial times, blackstrap molasses was the principal sweetener used in cooking. A rule of thumb is to use ½ cup of molasses for every cup of sugar called for in the recipe. According to *The Joy of Cooking*, you should also reduce other liquid that you may use by about ¼ cup for each ½ cup of molasses. In addition, add ½ teaspoon of baking soda for each ½ cup of molasses, and omit the baking powder.

POSSIBLE BENEFITS Both calcium and potassium are good for maintaining normal heart function, lowering blood pressure, and building strong bones.

Iron is essential for the formation of red cells. Iron deficiency can result in anemia, excess fatigue, and increased vulnerability to infection.

Blueberry

FACTS Eat these summer berries by the mouthful, throw them into fruit salad, bake them into muffins. Blueberry is high in pectin, a soluble form of dietary fiber that has been shown in many different studies to lower cholesterol. A cup of blueberries provides nearly a third of the RDA for vitamin C, and a fair amount of potassium, all at a mere 80 calories.

An old-time remedy for diarrhea, blueberries contain compounds called anthocyanosides, which help to control "the runs."

POSSIBLE BENEFITS Lowering cholesterol will significantly reduce your risk of developing coronary artery disease, which can lead to heart attack and stroke.

An antioxidant, vitamin C may help prevent the formation of plaque in the arteries, as well as many different forms of cancer. In addition, it increases your resistance against infection.

Potassium helps to maintain the normal fluid balance within the body, as well as normal heart function and blood pressure.

Bok Choy (Chinese Cabbage)

FACTS All cabbage is not the same: the varieties of cabbage that we commonly use to make coleslaw and stuffed cabbage are nowhere near as healthy as the kind of cabbage that is widely used in Chinese cooking. Western cabbage contains very little beta-carotene, the plant source of vitamin A. One cup of chopped bok choy contains nearly the entire RDA for beta-carotene, and that's not all. Bok choy is high in vitamin C, very rich in potassium, and also a good source of calcium—1 cup has roughly the same amount of calcium as in ½ cup of milk.

Like other members of the cruciferous family, bok choy contains indoles, phytochemicals that are believed to deactivate potent estrogens that can stimulate the growth of tumors, particularly in the breast. The National Cancer Institute is investigating the cruciferous family for its potential cancer-fighting properties.

POSSIBLE BENEFITS   Beta-carotene, an antioxidant, appears to protect against various forms of cancer and coronary artery disease.

Vitamin C, also an antioxidant, may help prevent cancer, and vitamin C is believed to help improve resistance against infection.

Calcium, which helps to build strong teeth and bones, is also important for normal blood pressure and heart function.

PERSONAL ADVICE   For a truly anticancer, heart-healthy, anticold and antiflu soup, sprinkle ½ cup raw bok choy in a bowl of hot chicken soup!

Broccoli

FACTS   Recently, broccoli has become a superstar of the vegetable world because it contains many compounds with important disease-fighting properties. Researchers H. Leon

Bradlow, Ph.D., and Jon J. Michnovicz, M.D., Ph.D., of the Institute for Hormone Research in New York, discovered that indoles, compounds found in cruciferous vegetables (broccoli, cabbage, kale, etc.), may be potential weapons against cancer. Indoles inactivate potent estrogens that can promote the growth of tumors in estrogen-sensitive cells, particularly those in the breast.

A research team at Johns Hopkins University School of Medicine discovered a compound in broccoli called sulforaphane that stimulates animal and human cells to produce cancer-fighting enzymes. Sulforaphane has also been found in kale, cauliflower, Brussels sprouts, carrots, and green onions.

Broccoli is also rich in beta-carotene, another well-known cancer fighter, as well as other essential vitamins and minerals. One broccoli spear contains about half the RDA for beta-carotene, more than twice the RDA for vitamin C, a hefty portion of potassium, and a fair amount of calcium, folic acid and selenium. It is also a good source of fiber.

POSSIBLE BENEFITS Indoles and sulforaphane may protect against various forms of cancer.

Beta-carotene is an antioxidant that protects the cell membrane against damage caused by free radicals. Oxidative damage is believed to be a factor in both cancer and heart disease.

Vitamin C is an antioxidant that protects against oxidative damage; it also helps the immune system fight against infection.

Potassium is essential for normal fluid balance in the cells. It also helps to normalize heart function and blood pressure.

Both calcium and folic acid protect against various forms of cancer.

Selenium protects against stroke and cancer.

Brown Rice

FACTS White rice is a perfect example of how food processing transforms a nutrient-rich, high-fiber food into a nutritional wasteland. In its natural state, rice (which is a brownish color) consists of a husk, bran, and germ. White rice is made by stripping the natural rice of nearly everything that is good, and then throwing in a few vitamins at the end to replace what has been lost. Brown rice, which goes through far less processing, is the whole grain without the outer husk. Because more of the good stuff is left in, brown rice has more vitamins and potassium than does white rice. More important, it has nearly twice the amount of fiber, which incidentally is one thing that is sorely lacking in most American diets. But don't get me wrong: don't eat brown rice just because it's good for you, eat it because it tastes good. As any rice aficionado will tell you, brown rice has a much richer flavor and more interesting texture. Once you start eating brown rice, you will not want to go back to its "washed-out" cousin.

POSSIBLE BENEFITS Rice bran is an excellent source of fiber. Fiber helps maintain bowel regularity and may help prevent certain forms of cancer.

Rice bran can lower cholesterol, which can reduce your risk of heart attack and stroke.

Brussels Sprouts

FACTS They look and taste like little cabbages, but they are big on nutrition. Like other members of the cruciferous family, such as broccoli and kale, Brussels sprouts contain a virtual arsenal of cancer-fighting compounds such as:

Indoles—chemicals that deactivate potent estrogens that can trigger tumor growth in estrogen-sensitive cells.

Sulforaphane—a chemical that stimulates animal and human cells to produce cancer-fighting enzymes.

Brussels sprouts contain an amazing 7.5 grams of fiber per one cup serving, making it one of the best vegetable sources of fiber. This vegetable is also packed with other important vitamins and minerals. A 1-cup serving contains a fair amount of beta-carotene and potassium, 150 percent of the RDA for vitamin C, and more than 10 percent of the RDA for iron and vitamin E.

POSSIBLE BENEFITS Sulforaphane helps the body rally its defenses against carcinogens.

Indoles may reduce your risk of developing breast cancer and other forms of cancer.

The high-fiber content helps maintain bowel regularity and protects against colon/rectal cancer.

All antioxidants—vitamins C, E, and beta-carotene—protect against cancer and coronary artery disease.

Buckwheat

FACTS Despite its name, buckwheat is not a kind of wheat, nor is it really even a grain. Buckwheat is actually the fruit of the *Fagopyrum* genus, which is related to rhubarb. The seed is dried and split—within it lies a kernel known as a groat, which is used much the same way as a grain. The unroasted kernel is pale—when roasted it turns a toasty brown color and is called kasha. Kasha, a mainstay of eastern European cuisine, is sold in most supermarkets and can be cooked like rice.

Buckwheat has all the goodness of whole grain—it is high in fiber and low in calories and fat. But it also has some important things that most grains lack. Buckwheat is rich in lysine, an amino acid that the body does not manufacture on its own and is not present in most grains. Diabetics take note: there is also some evidence that buckwheat may help keep glucose levels under control better than other carbohydrates. Recently, Indian scientists tested the effect of buckwheat on sugar metabolism. Students who were fed a buckwheat-rich diet showed an improvement in glucose tolerance, which means that their bodies were better able to utilize sugar from digested foods.

POSSIBLE BENEFITS Fiber helps promote bowel regularity and may help prevent various forms of cancer.

Buckwheat is wheat-free, and therefore a good grain alternative for people with wheat allergies.

Buckwheat enhances the body's ability to metabolize sugar, which may help prevent diabetes.

Buckwheat provides a more complete form of protein than many other grains, and therefore is particularly good for vegetarians.

Bulgur

FACTS Bulgur is wheat that has been parboiled, dried, and cracked. It is often used in Middle Eastern cooking in dishes such as tabouli and pilaf. At one time, bulgur enthusiasts had to buy this grain at an ethnic grocery or a specialty store, but today it is available in most supermarkets. Bulgur is not only an excellent source of fiber, but it is high in potassium and B vitamins. It also contains some iron and calcium. Although it is nutrient-rich, this grain is low in fat and calories.

POSSIBLE BENEFITS Fiber helps to promote bowel regularity and may prevent colon and rectal cancer.

Potassium helps to normalize high blood pressure, which reduces the risk of heart attack and stroke.

B vitamins in general are necessary for the conversion of food to energy.

PERSONAL ADVICE Try eating bulgur instead of white rice—it's tastier and a lot healthier.

Cantaloupe

FACTS If you're interested in reducing your risk of cancer and heart disease, make this melon an everyday part of your life. Half a cantaloupe more than satisfies your daily RDA of 5000 IU for beta-carotene. That's not all: it also provides an impressive 113 mg of vitamin C, nearly double the RDA for nonsmokers. An added bonus: 825 mg of potassium. And all at a modest 95 calories.

Cantaloupe is also a good source of fiber, weighing in at 1.8 grams per melon half.

POSSIBLE BENEFITS People who eat food rich in beta-carotene may be protected against developing certain forms of cancer, including lung, oral, colon, breast, cervical, and ovarian.

As a potent antioxidant, beta-carotene may protect against cataracts, which may be caused by the formation of free radicals which disrupt normal cellular growth.

The vitamin C in cantaloupe helps to prevent certain forms of cancer.

As antioxidants, both vitamin C and beta-carotene prevent the oxidation of LDL cholesterol that may contribute to the growth of plaque in the artery walls. This can lead to heart attack and stroke. Antioxidants such as beta-carotene and vitamin C are also believed to prevent premature aging.

The fiber content of cantaloupe helps maintain bowel regularity and prevent rectal cancer.

Carrot

FACTS Three carrots a day may be all it takes to keep you away from the cardiologist *and* the oncologist.

One raw carrot contains 13,500 IU of beta-carotene—more than 250 percent of the RDA. Beta-carotene is a potent antioxidant, which in addition to preventing the kind of cellular damage that can lead to cancer, also helps to prevent premature aging and cataracts.

Rich in fiber (the average carrot contains 2.3 grams of fiber), carrots contain calcium pectate, a type of soluble fiber that has been shown to reduce cholesterol. According to USDA researchers, two carrots a day may reduce total cholesterol levels by as much as 20 percent!

POSSIBLE BENEFITS May help reduce the risk of a wide range of cancers including lung, mouth, throat, stomach, intestine, bladder, prostate, and breast cancer.

By reducing cholesterol, carrots help to prevent coronary artery disease and stroke.

Cauliflower

FACTS Why is it that people who eat cruciferous vegetables, such as cauliflower, have lower rates of cancer than those who don't? It could be that cauliflower (like broccoli and Brussels sprouts) contains a compound called sulforaphane, which researchers at Johns Hopkins University School of Medicine recently learned can stimulate the production of cancer-fighting enzymes in the body. In other words, sulforaphane appears to help the body's cells ward off cancer-causing agents. But sulforaphane may not be the only reason why cauliflower may offer some protection against cancer. Cauliflower also contains a hefty dose of vitamin C, a potent antioxidant, as well as a good amount of potassium, fiber, and other essential vitamins and minerals.

POSSIBLE BENEFITS Contains compounds that may deactivate carcinogens.

Vitamin C may help to prevent various forms of cancer as well as coronary artery disease.

Potassium helps to maintain a normal fluid balance in the body as well as regulate heart function and blood pressure.

Fiber protects against colon/rectal cancer.

Celery

FACTS For more than 2000 years, celery has been used by Oriental healers to treat high blood pressure. Paradoxically, Western physicians have cautioned their patients to avoid celery because it is relatively high in sodium as compared with other vegetables—35 mg per stalk—which can actually increase blood pressure in susceptible individuals.

Researchers at the University of Chicago have recently discovered that the ancient healers may have been right. They found that a chemical in celery called 3-butylphthalide reduces blood pressure in laboratory rats by relaxing the smooth muscle lining of blood vessels. Once relaxed, the vessels dilate, allowing the blood to flow more freely throughout the body. When fed a dose of phthalide equivalent to what is found in four stalks of celery a day, the rats experienced a 13 percent drop in blood pressure and a 7 percent drop in cholesterol. If phthalide works the same way in humans—and there's no reason to think that it doesn't—it could explain why the Chinese often forego traditional blood pressure medication in favor of celery, which may provide the same benefit without any of the drug-induced side effects, such as dizziness or impotence.

Celery also contains compounds called psoralens which may help to prevent psoriasis, a chronic skin condition characterized by scaly red patches.

POSSIBLE BENEFITS Helps to prevent heart attack and stroke by reducing blood pressure and cholesterol.

May help to prevent psoriasis.

PERSONAL ADVICE If you're being treated for high blood pressure, don't discontinue your medication to try celery or any other remedy without first consulting with your physician. However, if you're a borderline hypertensive—that is, you have slightly higher than normal pressure and your physician is not sure whether or not you need medication—you may try eating four celery stalks daily for a week or so and see if it helps. Whatever you do, work closely with your physician or healer—do not dismiss high blood pressure as unimportant. Untreated, it can have devastating results.

Cherry

FACTS For many years, cherries were considered an unimportant fruit. Sure, they're naturally sweet and delicious, and at 5 calories per cherry, a better snack choice than a lot of other highly sugared, fat-laden foods. However, their numbers are unimpressive: they offer little in the way of vitamins C or A and are lower in nutrients than many other fruits. So, how did the "unimportant" cherry end up on a list of "Hot Hundred" foods? Recently, researchers have discovered that cherries are one of a handful of fruits that contain a powerful compound known as ellagic acid. Ellagic acid is important because it counteracts synthetic and naturally occurring carcinogens, preventing them from wreaking havoc on healthy cells and turning them into cancerous ones.

POSSIBLE BENEFITS By inactivating carcinogens, the ellagic acid may help prevent cancer.

Chicken Soup

FACTS When I was studying to be a pharmacist, my classmates and I used to snicker at relatives who said that their home-brewed cures were as effective as our dazzling arsenal of chemical wonders. It seemed outrageous to us that something as simple as chicken soup could be as useful a treatment for the common cold as our battery of antihistamines and decongestants. As it turned out, your grandmother was right! Researchers at Mount Sinai Hospital in Miami Beach discovered that chicken soup works better than any other liquid in breaking up the mucus and congestion of a cold. Pulmonary researchers gave patients cold water, hot water and chicken soup, and each time measured the clearance rate of nasal mucus. Chicken soup won, no contest. In addition, researchers believe that chicken soup may be a mild antibiotic, that is, it helps the body to fight infection.

POSSIBLE BENEFITS Helps to loosen nasal mucus and fight respiratory infections.

PERSONAL ADVICE For a stuffy nose, sit over a hot bowl of chicken soup and inhale the vapor for five minutes before eating. This "Jewish Penicillin" works as well as many over-the-counter cold medications, without the unpleasant side effects such as drowsiness and irritation of the nasal passages.

Chili Peppers (Cayenne or Capsicum)

FACTS Their botanical name, *Capsicum frutescens,* is derived from the Greek *kapto,* "I bite," and bite they do. When

Columbus first took a bite out of a red chili pepper in the West Indies, he thought that he had found a different plant source for black pepper, a highly valued spice. Despite their stinging sensation, chilis are not at all related to the *Piper nigrum* plant, but the name "pepper" stuck anyway.

Chilis contain a compound called capsaicin, which gives them their unique sting. Since ancient times, chilis have been used externally by healers to relieve pain. Recently, scientists learned that capsaicin stimulates certain nerve cells to release a chemical called substance P, which sends pain signals throughout the nervous system. Capsaicin quickly depletes the cells of substance P, thus temporarily blocking their ability to transmit anymore pain impulses. Capsaicin ointment is now used to alleviate the pain of arthritis and shingles. A nose spray of capsaicin is being studied as a possible treatment for cluster headaches, a particularly painful condition.

If you bite into a chili pepper, you will feel a rush of heat that burns the mouth, but paradoxically may soothe the nerves. Taken internally, capsaicin triggers the release of endorphins in the brain, which has a pain-relieving effect similar to morphine.

Chili peppers are good for the body as well as the soul. One pepper contains a full day's supply of beta-carotene and nearly twice the RDA for vitamin C. Chilis have been shown to cut cholesterol in animal studies. Rats fed capsaicin along with a diet low in saturated fat lost weight and lowered their triglycerides. It also lowered LDL or bad cholesterol in male rats. Recently, two scientists in Connecticut discovered that chilis may contain a previously unrecognized antioxidant, which means that this strange food may also protect against cancer and heart disease. Scientists at the Max Planck Institute found that chili peppers can prevent blood clots by extending blood coagulation time.

Chilis may also help keep you slim by speeding up your metabolism. After eating hot peppers, you tend to sweat, a sign that your metabolism is shifting into high gear.

UCLA researcher Dr. Irving Ziment recommends using chilis to help alleviate the symptoms of the common cold. Dr. Ziment says chilis can help break up congestion and keep the airways clear.

Hot spicy foods contain liberal amounts of cayenne or capsicum, which stimulates the production of gastric juices, improves metabolism, and even helps relieve gas.

POSSIBLE BENEFITS Beta-carotene and vitamin C can protect against various forms of cancer and cardiovascular disease.

Chili peppers are good decongestants and can help prevent bronchitis.

Chili peppers can also relieve discomfort caused by the common cold and may help control pain.

Chili peppers may help cut cholesterol and triglycerides and decrease LDL or bad cholesterol.

Chili peppers may improve circulation, which protects against heart attack and stroke.

CAUTION Chili peppers can aggravate hemorrhoids and existing ulcers. However, contrary to popular belief, spicy food does not promote stomach distress, cause ulcers, or harm a normal stomach. In addition, wash your hands before touching your face or eyes after cutting a chili pepper; otherwise, it could be irritating.

PERSONAL ADVICE To cool down after eating a hot chili pepper, drink a glass of milk. Casein, a protein in milk, counteracts capsaicin.

Cinnamon

FACTS You may think of it as something to spice up a hot toddy or flavor a coffee cake, but people in the know are making cinnamon a regular part of their lives. Take Richard Anderson, Ph.D., of the USDA's Human Nutrition Center, who makes it a point to sprinkle a liberal amount of cinnamon on his morning oatmeal. Dr. Anderson knows what he is doing. He is one of a handful of scientific researchers who are investigating the potential health benefits of cinnamon and other spices. Recent animal studies show that cinnamon greatly enhances the ability of insulin to metabolize glucose, that is, it can help control blood sugar levels. Obviously, this is good news for diabetics whose problem stems from their inability to produce enough insulin to use food properly. Although there have not been any formal trials involving humans, Dr. Anderson says that many diabetics have told him that eating ¼ teaspoon or so a day of cinnamon has had a beneficial effect on their blood sugar levels.

POSSIBLE BENEFITS May help insulin to work more efficiently, thus enhancing the body's ability to convert glucose into energy.

By helping to control diabetes, may help to prevent coronary artery disease and high blood pressure.

Cod

FACTS The people of Iceland can boast the longest life span of any other nationality in the Western world. Do Icelanders owe their longevity to the fact that they consume more of this fish than anyone else? While we're wolfing down cheeseburgers and fries, Icelanders are eating cod, and lots of it. But even a lot of cod won't make you fat or clog your arteries. Cod is incredibly low in saturated fat and calories. One 4-ounce serving has a mere 118 calories and a minute 37 mg of cholesterol. An added bonus: as fish go, cod is relatively pollutant-free since it is both low in fat (which stores contaminants) and is caught offshore, away from polluted rivers and streams.

POSSIBLE BENEFITS   Eating low-fat food such as cod can help lower cholesterol and reduce your risk of heart disease and certain forms of cancer.

Corn

FACTS   Christopher Columbus brought corn from the New World back to Spain, where it was received with wild enthusiasm. For thousands of years, corn has been a staple among the Indians of Mexico, where incidentally cholesterol levels are low and heart disease is a rarity. Whether or not corn can take all the credit for the low rate of heart disease among these tribes is a matter of debate. However, no one can dispute that corn is good for you. One sweet, cooked corn on the cob is a mere 90 calories and a hefty 2.4 grams of dietary fiber. Corn also contains a generous amount of potassium and a touch of vitamin A.

POSSIBLE BENEFITS   Fiber helps prevent constipation, and may reduce the risk of developing various forms of cancer.

Potassium helps to maintain normal blood pressure and heart function, which reduces the risk of heart attack and stroke.

Cranberry

FACTS Several years ago, a friend asked me what she could do to prevent cystitis, a painful but common urinary tract infection that has a tendency to recur from time to time. She expected me to prescribe a regimen of high-potency vitamins and minerals, with a few herbs thrown in for good measure. Instead, much to her surprise, I told her to drink a glass or two of cranberry juice daily. Although she was skeptical, she followed my advice. She has not been bothered by a urinary tract infection since.

Ten years ago, when I first advised my friend to try cranberry juice, scientists were puzzled as to why the juice of this particular berry seemed to ward off urinary tract infections. Some believed that cranberry changed the pH of the urine in such a way that it killed bacteria. However, as logical as that explanation may seem, it is not the real reason. In order to understand how cranberry works, you need to understand just what causes the infection in the first place. The culprit is the *E. coli* bacterium, which has a tendency to stick to the walls of the urinary tract, the path the urine takes when it leaves the kidneys, travels to the urethra, and is excreted through the vaginal opening. In 1988, researchers at the Alliance City Hospital in Ohio discovered that cranberry juice had a "Teflon effect" on *E. coli* bacteria—it somehow prevented the troublesome bacteria from sticking to the endothelial cells of the urinary tract, and as a result, it was flushed out of the body through the urine.

POSSIBLE BENEFITS Can help prevent urinary tract infections from recurring or occurring in the first place.

PERSONAL ADVICE The best cranberry juice is the non-sweetened, 100 percent pure juice that is sold primarily in natural food stores. Cranberry juice concentrate is now available in capsule form as a food supplement.

Although cranberry juice is a wonderful way of helping to prevent urinary tract infections, if you think that you already have an infection, see your physician for further treatment. If untreated, these infections can lead to serious complications including kidney damage. Symptoms include burning upon urination, frequent urge to urinate, as well as abdominal pain and fever. It is especially important not to ignore these symptoms during pregnancy or to try to treat them yourself.

Cucumber

FACTS Here's one food that you can eat to your heart's content. At a scant 14 calories per cup, cucumber is a godsend for a dieter with a bad case of the "munchies." Cucumber is also good for your heart—this crisp and refreshing vegetable contains compounds called sterols, which have been shown to lower cholesterol in animals.

POSSIBLE BENEFITS May help protect against coronary artery disease by reducing cholesterol.

PERSONAL ADVICE The heaviest concentration of sterols is in the skin of the cucumber. Therefore, you should not remove the peel before eating. Unfortunately, cucumbers can be heavily waxed to help make them shiny and preserve their moisture. You can remove some of the wax residue, but not all, by scrubbing the cucumber well in cool water with a brush. If you want to avoid residue altogether, buy organically grown cucumbers.

Curry

FACTS Although curry is often sold as a single spice, it is actually a combination of spices. A typical curry includes turmeric (the spice that gives it its golden color), cinnamon, garlic, ginger, cardamom, coriander, cumin, as well as other spices.

Before refrigeration, many curry spices were used to prevent food from going rancid. Back then, no one knew exactly why these spices worked. Today we know that many spices are actually potent antioxidants, that is, they prevent the formation of free radicals that can cause damage to normal cells as well as promote aging. We also know that some curry spices have an antibiotic effect. They can help fight bacteria that may cause food poisoning.

Curry spices have also been shown to lower cholesterol and prevent the formation of blood clots.

A recent study sponsored by the USDA shows that turmeric enhances the ability of insulin to metabolize glucose, which may help control diabetes.

Several Indian studies have shown that curry spices have an anti-inflammatory effect on the body.

For centuries, curry has been used by Indian healers to aid digestion.

POSSIBLE BENEFITS The antioxidants in curry may help prevent certain forms of cancer, as well as protect against premature aging.

By lowering cholesterol and preventing blood clots, curry may help protect against heart attack and stroke.

Curry may help diabetics control blood sugar levels.

By preventing inflammation, curry may help reduce the aches and pains associated with arthritis.

Dandelion Greens

FACTS To gardeners, they're just troublesome weeds, but to healers through the ages, the greens and roots from this plant are highly prized, and for several good reasons. First, dandelion greens are an excellent source of beta-carotene and vitamin C, two vitamins that many Americans lack in their diets.

Second, there is growing evidence that dandelions may have a beneficial effect on liver function. For centuries, herbal healers have used dandelions as a treatment for liver ailments and an overall liver tonic. Today we know that this plant is rich in lecithin, which researchers are now investigating as a possible treatment for cirrhosis of the liver. In addition, there are other compounds in dandelions that have been shown to stimulate bile production, which can help the liver do its job more efficiently.

POSSIBLE BENEFITS A potent antioxidant, beta-carotene helps protect against heart disease and various forms of cancer.

Vitamin C, also an antioxidant, protects against heart disease and cancer and helps boost the immune system.

Eggplant

FACTS Despite its name, eggplant is not related to the egg at all; it is so-named because the white variety of this vegetable resembles an egg in appearance. Most people, however, are familiar with the shiny, purple eggplant which is sold in most supermarkets and greengroceries. Eggplant is a member of the Solanaceae family (along with pepper and tomato) which is being investigated by the National Cancer Institute for its potential as a cancer fighter. Solanaceae vegetables are packed with important phytochemicals that have been shown to block the cancer formation process. For example, eggplant contains terpenes which may deactivate steroidal hormones that can promote certain types of tumors, and may also prevent oxidative damage that can make a cell susceptible to cancerous growth. Eggplant is also a heart-healthy food: it provides a fair amount of potassium, which helps to normalize blood pressure, and is extremely low in fat and calories.

POSSIBLE BENEFITS May help prevent the initiation and spread of different types of cancerous growth.

By regulating blood pressure and heart function, helps to prevent heart attack and stroke.

PERSONAL ADVICE Many people prepare eggplant by breading it and frying it in oil. Unfortunately, eggplant soaks up oil like a sponge—"oven fry" breaded eggplant instead, using a small amount of heart-healthy oil such as canola.

Flounder (Sole)

FACTS Flounder and sole are close relatives and it is nearly impossible to tell the difference. In many fish markets, they are sold interchangeably. The only true sole is Dover sole, imported from Europe—it is expensive and often difficult to come by. Flounder and sole are mild-tasting, flat fish that can be found in the Atlantic and Pacific and on the Gulf coasts. Lemon sole is caught in Atlantic waters; gray sole and other smaller, delicately flavored varieties are caught in Pacific waters. No matter what it's called, flounder is good for you. A 3-ounce serving is a mere 80 calories with only 1 gram of fat, and virtually no saturated fat. These are fantastic numbers considering that a hamburger made from a lean cut of meat is 230 calories and 16 grams of fat!

POSSIBLE BENEFITS Low-fat foods help reduce cholesterol; elevated cholesterol is a leading risk factor for heart attack and stroke.

Low-fat foods also reduce the risk of various forms of cancer.

Garlic

FACTS This hot food of the twenty-first century dates back to the time of the pyramids. Garlic is now at the top of the list of foods being investigated by the National Cancer Institute as a potential weapon against many different forms of cancer. Although the scientific community has recently focused its attention on this herb, garlic has a rich and illustrious history as a healing food. The Egyptians worshipped it, and placed clay models of garlic bulbs in the tomb of Tutankhamen. Hippocrates, the father of modern medicine, used garlic vapors to treat cervical cancer. In the Middle Ages, monks chewed on garlic cloves to protect themselves against plague. During World War II, when antibiotics were scarce, garlic poultices were placed on wounds to prevent infection.

There are more than 1000 serious studies that have been performed on garlic in recent years. From these studies we know that allicin, a compound in fresh garlic, has antibiotic and antifungal properties. Researchers are also beginning to unravel the complex chemistry of garlic. Among some of their more important findings:

♦ Diallyl sulfide (DAS), a component of garlic oil, has been shown to inactivate potent carcinogens in animal studies. DAS reduced the metabolism of nitrosamine, a particularly lethal naturally occurring carcinogen, by the liver. It also suppresses the growth of tumors.
♦ Garlic compounds stimulate the formation of gluta-thione, an amino acid that detoxifies foreign materials and is a potent antioxidant.

Renowned first-century physician Dioscorides wrote that garlic "clears the arteries and opens the mouths of veins." Researchers are confirming that garlic is good for cardiovascular health. Several studies have shown that garlic can lower cholesterol—specifically LDL or "bad" cholesterol—in animals and humans. In fact, garlic may work as well as some anticholesterol drugs such as clofibrate, without the unpleasant side effects. Scientist Eric Block also discovered a compound in garlic called ajoene, a natural blood thinner, which helps prevent the formation of blood clots.

Garlic is tricky to use, however, because it is highly unstable—its chemistry changes depending on how it's used. When crushed, it releases chemicals called thiosulfinates, including allicin, which are responsible for its pungent odor. If you steam or cook it, you release different chemicals. Scientists disagree as to which form of garlic offers the best protection against cancer, and hopefully, NCI researchers will come up with some concrete answers. However, any form of garlic is believed to be effective in lowering cholesterol and improving circulation.

POSSIBLE BENEFITS May deactivate carcinogens, thus preventing the growth of cancerous tumors.

By lowering cholesterol, helps prevent heart attack and stroke.

By preventing the formation of blood clots, helps promote good circulation and protects against heart attack and stroke.

PERSONAL ADVICE I prefer stir-frying or baking garlic to eating it raw. It goes down a lot easier! Elephant garlic has a much milder odor. If you can't stand garlic breath, supplements of aged, raw, odorless garlic are available. Take them with an internal breath freshener made from parsley seed oil.

Ginger

FACTS For centuries, Chinese healers have been using ginger as an antinauseant for motion sickness, morning sickness, and general stomach upset. Now Western physicians have begun to take a second look at his herb. A case in point is a recent article in *Anaesthesia*, which describes a novel way to treat postoperative vomiting and nausea that are typical after procedures involving general anesthesia. Sixty women who had been given general anesthesia for gynecological surgery were divided into two groups. One group was given a well-known antinauseant. The other was given ginger capsules. The group on ginger appeared to experience fewer symptoms than those on the antinausea drug and, in fact, were able to recuperate without any additional medication for stomach upset. I have also heard of cases in which ginger tea made from fresh root was used quite successfully to help alleviate the nausea typical of chemotherapy.

Ginger is also being investigated by the National Cancer Institute for its potential anticancer properties.

`POSSIBLE BENEFITS` Ginger is a natural way to help relieve nausea. It is particularly useful for people suffering from drug-induced nausea, since it will not interact in a negative way with their other medication.

Ginger is a safe remedy for morning sickness, since it will not harm the fetus.

Ginger may help prevent certain forms of cancer.

`PERSONAL ADVICE` The Japanese eat thin slices of ginger with sushi. If you don't want to eat it straight, try brewing a tea. Slice some ginger root, put it in a tea ball and place in a teapot. Pour boiling hot water over the tea ball and let it sit for ten minutes. Sweeten with honey or drink it straight.

Grape

`FACTS` There's been a lot of publicity lately about how wine drinkers have fewer heart attacks and live longer than teetotalers. Wine's protective effect on the cardiovascular system has been attributed to a compound called resveratrol, which Japanese researchers have recently shown could prevent atherosclerosis in animals. Now a scientist from Cornell University, Leroy Creasy, Ph.D., has found that red grape juice has as much resveratrol as many wines, and, in some cases, even more. Better yet, grape juice won't get you drunk and it's safe for children.

According to Dr. Creasy's study, there is very little resveratrol in white wine, in white grape juice, or in green grapes themselves. However, there are still some very compelling reasons to eat grapes of any color. First, they are a good source of ellagic acid, which is believed to be a strong anti-cancer compound. Second, grapes are also rich in boron, a mineral that may help postmenopausal women maintain higher blood levels of estrogen.

POSSIBLE BENEFITS Grapes may help prevent heart attack and stroke by reducing cholesterol.

Ellagic acid, a compound in grapes, has been shown to counteract carcinogens.

Boron, a trace mineral found in grapes, may help prevent osteoporosis or bone thinning in older women by maintaining higher levels of estrogen. (Estrogen is essential for calcium absorption.)

Grapefruit

FACTS If you don't eat at least one grapefruit a day, you're missing a lot. First, this remarkable fruit is one of nature's best cholesterol fighters. The pulpy membrane that separates the individual segments is full of pectin, a form of soluble fiber that seems to melt away cholesterol. Consider a recent study at the University of Florida College of Medicine in which people with high cholesterol were given grapefruit pectin supplements. Within 16 weeks, the group's cholesterol dropped an average 7.6 percent, with the "bad" LDL cholesterol declining by more than 10 percent.

But this is just the beginning of the grapefruit story. Grapefruit, like its other citrus cousins, contains limonene, a citrus oil which has been shown to significantly reduce the growth of mammary tumors in laboratory rats. In addition, limonene inhibited the formation of subsequent tumors. No wonder that the National Cancer Institute (NCI) is spending millions of dollars investigating the cancer-fighting potential of limonene and other citrus oils.

The NCI is taking a close look at citrus fruits such as grapefruit because they are loaded with biologically active substances that may help prevent cancer. Citrus contains flavonoids, potent antioxidants that may help prevent the spread of cancer. In addition, citrus has phenolics which may help the body produce substances to detoxify carcinogens such as nitrosamine.

Grapefruit is also loaded with vitamin C. One half grapefruit provides 41 mg of vitamin C, two thirds of the RDA for nonsmokers.

Ruby red grapefruit offers an additional bonus: it is rich in a carotenoid called lycopene. Lycopene may offer protection against cervical, bladder, and pancreatic cancer.

POSSIBLE BENEFITS   By lowering cholesterol, the pectin in grapefruit helps prevent against heart attack and stroke.

Lycopene, limonene, and the other biologically active substances in grapefruit may help protect against various forms of cancer.

The vitamin C in grapefruit, a potent antioxidant, may help prevent heart disease by preventing the oxidation of LDL or "bad" cholesterol, which may lead to plaque deposits in the artery walls.

Vitamin C has been shown to lessen the severity of colds.

PERSONAL ADVICE Throw out your grapefruit knife! By just eating the segments, you're throwing away one of the healthiest parts of the grapefruit—the pectin. For maximum benefit, eat the whole fruit.

Also, as wonderful as grapefruit may be, contrary to popular myth (à la the Grapefruit Diet) it does not help you lose weight. There are people who believe that even if they gorge on a diet high in fat and calories, eating grapefruit on top of everything else will help them melt the pounds away. Unfortunately, this is not true. However, grapefruit can help you shed pounds if you eat it instead of high-fat dessert.

Green Tea

FACTS For centuries, Japanese parents have advised their children to drink green tea after eating a sweet. Researchers at the University of California at Berkeley recently learned that flavor compounds in Japanese tea can kill *Streptococcus mutans,* bacteria that are responsible for the initiation of cavities.

Green tea may not only prevent cavities but also help fight against heart disease. Green tea is rich in catechins, substances that have been shown to lower cholesterol in laboratory animals. Other studies show that catechins may have antioxidant properties and may also help the body to retain vitamin C.

Green tea may also protect against cancer. A recent study performed at Rutgers University noted that a compound in green tea that was added to the animals' drinking water inhibited the growth of skin tumors on mice. Hirota Fujiki, a Japanese researcher, is quoted as saying, "We would like to think drinking green tea may be one of the most practical cancer preventions at this moment."

POSSIBLE BENEFITS May help to prevent dental caries and gum disease.

By reducing cholesterol, may help to prevent coronary artery disease and stroke.

Catechins have antioxidant properties which may help prevent lung and skin cancer and heart disease by protecting cells against damage by free radicals.

CAUTION Studies have shown that massive doses of catechins can be toxic. However, a cup or two a day appears to be both safe and beneficial.

PERSONAL ADVICE Real green tea is found in Oriental markets or health food stores in bulk or in tea bags. Supermarkets usually sell black tea, which may not offer the same benefits. In the central Japanese area of Shizuoka-ken where green tea is produced, and people drink far greater amounts than in other parts of Japan, there is a much reduced incidence of cancer. More research is needed, but I would recommend your drinking green tea.

Guava

FACTS This sweet tropical fruit contains more than twice the vitamin C of an orange: one guava provides nearly 300 percent of the RDA for ascorbic acid. Guava is also one of nature's best sources of dietary fiber and has a good amount of beta-carotene and potassium. What guava lacks is calories and fat—one fruit weighs in at under 50 calories.

POSSIBLE BENEFITS Vitamin C and beta-carotene are potent antioxidants which may prevent the kind of cellular damage that leads to cancerous mutations. Antioxidants may also help to prevent the formation of plaque in the arteries, which can cause atherosclerosis.

Vitamin C may decrease the body's susceptibility to infection.

Potassium helps maintain normal blood pressure and heart function.

Kale

FACTS We may believe that we "discovered" the wonders of this terrific vegetable; however, kale has been grown for food since 200 B.C. The leaves and the stem of this plant are edible (and quite tasty). A member of the illustrious cruciferous family, kale contains cancer-fighting compounds such as sulforaphane and indoles. It also contains an amazing amount of beta-carotene, the plant form of vitamin A—one cup of kale has nearly 10,000 IU of vitamin A, almost twice the RDA. Kale also has nearly a day's supply of vitamin C and vitamin E and even some calcium (about 10 percent of the RDA). To round out a nearly perfect picture, kale is also high in fiber and potassium.

POSSIBLE BENEFITS Sulforaphane stimulates the body to produce cancer-fighting enzymes.

Indoles deactivate potent estrogens that stimulate tumor growth.

Antioxidants beta-carotene, vitamin C, and vitamin E aid in proper immune system function and protect against many different forms of cancer and heart disease.

Calcium and potassium help maintain normal blood pressure.

Fiber protects against colon/rectal cancer.

Kiwifruit

FACTS Native to New Zealand, this fruit is bursting with vitamin C—one kiwi has 120 percent of the RDA for this important vitamin. Kiwi is also low in calories (45 per fruit) and has a respectable amount of fiber and potassium. Better yet, this fruit is absolutely delicious and is terrific in fruit salad or eaten alone.

POSSIBLE BENEFITS Vitamin C may help prevent certain types of cancer and heart disease.

Vitamin C may also give the immune system ammunition to fight off viruses such as the one that causes the common cold. Although it can't cure a cold, there is evidence that it may shorten the duration and severity of a cold.

Fiber helps to maintain bowel regularity and may protect against rectal and colon cancer.

Potassium helps maintain the proper fluid balance in the body's cells, and helps maintain normal heart function and blood pressure.

Kohlrabi

`FACTS` Kohlrabi, a cross between a turnip and a cabbage, can be steamed and served hot as a side dish, or sliced cold and cut into a salad. Kohlrabi is very high in vitamin C— one cup of cooked kohlrabi contains 150 percent of the RDA. It is also abundant in potassium and contains more than 10 percent of the RDA for vitamin E.

Kohlrabi (along with broccoli, kale, cabbage) is a member of the cruciferous family, which is being investigated by the National Cancer Institute for its potential cancer-fighting properties.

`POSSIBLE BENEFITS` Vitamin C and vitamin E are antioxidants, which may prevent the formation of cancerous tumors.

Vitamin C helps the body ward off infection.

Antioxidants may also play a role in preventing plaque deposits in arteries, which can lead to coronary artery disease.

`PERSONAL ADVICE` Try to buy young kohlrabi bulbs, they're more tender and don't need to be peeled. (You must peel the older bulbs because they're very tough.)

Lemon

`FACTS` Lemon, like other members of the citrus family, is packed with vitamin C, which is good for everything from cancer to the common cold. No wonder that the National Cancer Institute has targeted the citrus family as one of the food groups that has the greatest lifesaving potential.

One lemon contains 30 mg of vitamin C, half the amount of this vitamin recommended for nonsmokers. Lemon is also rich in flavonoids, biologically active substances that perform many different beneficial roles in the body, often in conjunction with vitamin C. Some flavonoids are potent antioxidants; others help regulate enzymes that may promote the growth of tumors. As with other citrus fruits, lemons also contain terpenes, substances that control the production of cholesterol, and set in motion a chain reaction that blocks the action of certain carcinogens.

Lemons are also a good source of limonene, a citrus oil that has been shown to thwart the growth of cancerous tumors in animals.

POSSIBLE BENEFITS Vitamin C is a potent antioxidant that helps prevent cancer and increases the body's ability to fight off infection.

Limonene may help shrink cancerous tumors and prevent their regrowth.

Flavonoids are believed to help the body fight off viruses, alleviate allergic reactions, and even prevent certain forms of cancer.

Terpenes help control cholesterol and stimulate enzymes that prevent carcinogens from destroying healthy cells.

PERSONAL ADVICE As good as a lemon may be for you, it does taste sour—not too many people can suffer their way through a whole lemon. Therefore, I advise people to use lemon juice as a seasoning whenever possible. Sprinkle it on fresh vegetables, fruits, and in tea. Make fresh lemonade or lemon ices in the summer.

Lentil

FACTS In the Old Testament, Esau sold his birthright to his brother for a bowl of lentil soup—I'm not sure who got the best of the bargain. Like other legumes, lentils are a terrific source of soluble and insoluble fiber: ½ cup serving has 3.7 grams of dietary fiber. Lentils are also high in protein (although it is not a complete protein) and low in fat and calories. Lentils are exceptionally rich in folic acid and also contain a healthy dose of potassium, iron, and copper.

Lentils (also other beans, grains, and seeds) contain compounds called phytates which appear to ward off cancerous changes in cells. According to one study, mice on a high-fat diet were given injections of carcinogens to induce cancerous changes in the breast and colon. Some of the mice were also given megadoses of calcium and iron, which appeared to promote the growth of cancerous tumors. However, when scientists added phytates to the diet of the mice, the onset of cancer was dramatically reduced.

POSSIBLE BENEFITS Soluble fiber has been shown to reduce blood cholesterol levels, which reduces the risk of diabetes and cardiovascular disease.

Insoluble fiber promotes bowel regularity by speeding up the food passage through the digestive tract. This form of fiber is believed to reduce the risk of developing colon cancer.

Folic acid helps to prevent neural tube defects in the fetus, and protects against various forms of cancer and heart disease.

Iron helps to prevent anemia and is especially important for menstruating and pregnant women.

Copper may help prevent dangerous soluble clots which can cause heart attacks and stroke.

Lettuce (Romaine)

FACTS   When the National Cancer Institute says that Americans should eat more dark green, leafy vegetables, lettuce is one of the first foods that come to mind. However, all lettuce is not the same. Romaine is head and shoulders above the rest. The numbers tell the story. One cup of romaine lettuce contains 1060 IU of beta-carotene, about 20 percent of the RDA. You'd have to eat a whole head of iceberg or Boston lettuce to get that same amount of beta-carotene. Romaine also has twice the fiber (1 gram) and potassium (180 mg) of iceberg.

POSSIBLE BENEFITS   Beta-carotene may help prevent many different forms of cancer as well as heart disease.

Fiber helps maintain normal bowel regularity as well as prevent cancers of the colon and rectum.

PERSONAL ADVICE   Don't negate the health benefits of lettuce by dousing it in a high-fat salad dressing. Use low-fat commercial dressings, or better yet, squeeze some lemon juice and a small amount of olive oil on your salad.

Mackerel

FACTS   In terms of nutrition, mackerel is a superfish. It is one of the richest food sources of omega-3 fatty acids—2.1 grams per 4-ounce serving. According to the National Heart and Lung Institute, just 1 gram of omega-3 fatty acids daily may reduce the risk of cardiovascular disease in men by as much as 40 percent. (Although the studies were done on men, it doesn't necessarily mean that women will not reap the same benefits.) In addition to being "heart healthy," this fish has a lot of other good things to offer. Mackerel has more than 10 percent of the RDA for calcium, and is a good source of vitamin D, which aids in the absorption of calcium. It is also rich in antioxidants vitamin A and E. To round out the picture, mackerel is packed with B vitamins: mackerel is an excellent source of niacin, and a good source of thiamine, B_{12}, and riboflavin.

POSSIBLE BENEFITS   Omega-3 fatty acids:

- May reduce cholesterol in people with elevated cholesterol, and can lower blood pressure in people with high blood pressure, which lowers their risk of developing coronary artery disease or having a stroke
- May lower triglycerides in patients with high triglycerides (triglycerides over 190 mg/dl put women at risk of heart attack; over 400 mg/dl increases the risk for men); reduce the risk of blood clots which could lead to stroke and heart attack
- May reduce inflammation in patients with psoriasis, ulcerative colitis, arthritis, lupus, and asthma
- May inhibit the growth of cancerous tumors in animals
- Are present in breast milk, and essential for normal brain and eye development

Calcium and vitamin D are essential for strong teeth and bones.

Beta-carotene and vitamin E can help prevent oxidative damage to cells that can initiate cancer. They also protect against heart attack and stroke.

B-complex is necessary for the normal functioning of the nervous system, as well as many other important jobs in the body. A deficiency in B vitamins can result in fatigue, depression, and a weakened immune system.

Mango

FACTS If you're looking to get more fiber and vitamins into your life, try eating a mango. This yellowish-red tropical fruit is simply bursting with beta-carotene, the plant form of vitamin A. One mango has more than 8000 IU of beta-carotene; that's over 150 percent of the RDA. The average mango also provides nearly a day's supply of vitamin C and a good amount of potassium. In the fiber arena, mango is a true superstar—one fruit has nearly 7 grams of dietary fiber.

POSSIBLE BENEFITS Beta-carotene may protect against many different forms of cancer and atherosclerosis, which can lead to heart attack and stroke.

Vitamin C, a potent antioxidant, may help to prevent cancer and heart disease and helps the body fight against infection.

Fiber helps to maintain bowel regularity and protects against colon and rectal cancer.

Milk, Nonfat

FACTS The Physicians' Committee for Responsible Medicine recently made quite a stir by warning parents that cow's milk can be dangerous to their children's health. The group contended that milk can cause serious allergic reactions in many children and may also trigger diabetes. There is some truth to these allegations. Although it is relatively rare, some children are allergic to milk and should not drink it. There is also some evidence—although it is hardly conclusive—that a protein in milk may destroy insulin-producing cells, thereby contributing to insulin-dependent diabetes in children. However, even if milk does affect insulin production, this problem would only affect children with a genetic predisposition to develop diabetes, a very small percentage of the population.

In addition, many adults are lactose-intolerant, that is, they have difficulty digesting milk.

Given all of these negatives, how did milk wind up in the Hot Hundred? I believe that for the majority of children and certainly many adults, milk is not only safe but actually good for them. Milk is an excellent source of calcium, riboflavin, vitamin D, and phosphorus. Although whole milk is high in fat, skim milk (nonfat) and milk with 1 percent fat content (2 grams of fat per cup) are healthy alternatives. Vitamin D is added to milk to help aid in calcium absorption.

Calcium is important for people of all ages, but recent studies suggest that it is especially important for children. Researchers in the Framingham Children's Study monitored the calcium intake of 80 preschoolers. According to the study, the children with the highest intake of calcium-rich foods had the lowest blood pressure. Studies in adults also show that people who have the highest calcium intakes have the lowest blood pressure.

Calcium is also an essential mineral for girls and women. According to the Surgeon General's Report on Nutrition and Health, the median daily calcium intake for girls between the ages of 12 and 14 was roughly 790 mg, nowhere near the 1200 mg RDA. The report notes that chronically low calcium intake during adolescence may hinder peak bone mass growth, which may contribute to osteoporosis later in life. Considering the virtual epidemic of osteoporosis among older women in this country, parents should be especially vigilant about their daughters' calcium intake.

Of course, there are other foods that are rich in calcium, such as broccoli, kale, tofu, and canned salmon with bones. However, a child would have to eat roughly 4 to 6 cups of vegetables to get the same amount of calcium found in 2 cups of milk, and for many children, that may be hard to swallow. In addition, vegetables contain phytates, substances that may interfere with the absorption of minerals such as calcium. Therefore, milk is still the best way to get calcium into kids.

POSSIBLE BENEFITS Calcium is essential for strong bones and teeth. It helps regulate normal blood pressure and heart function.

Vitamin D and phosphorus work with calcium to build strong bones.

PERSONAL ADVICE If you are lactose-intolerant, try eating yogurt. It's easier on the stomach and is also a terrific source of calcium. There are also some new lactose-free dairy products that may go down a bit easier. For a low-fat calcium boost, try using buttermilk in your baking. The buttermilk available today is a lot different than it was in the past. Old-fashioned buttermilk was a thick liquid left over after the milk was churned into butter. It was high in both fat and calories. Today, buttermilk is made from 1 percent low-fat milk with added bacterial cultures. It adds a fluffy and moist consistency to foods such as muffins and pancakes, at a very reasonable 99 calories per cup.

Mustard Greens

FACTS If you've never tasted these succulent greens, you're in for a treat. Mustard greens are not only delicious but packed with an arsenal of nutrients to combat cancer and heart disease. A member of the cruciferous family, mustard greens contain indoles, compounds that deactivate potent estrogens that stimulate the growth of tumors. This vegetable is also filled with important vitamins and minerals. One cup of cooked mustard greens provides nearly 100 percent of the RDA for beta-carotene, 50 percent of the RDA for vitamin C, and more than 10 percent of a day's supply of iron and calcium.

POSSIBLE BENEFITS Cruciferous vegetables contain cancer-fighting compounds.

Beta-carotene may prevent various forms of cancer and heart disease.

An antioxidant, vitamin C may protect against cancer and heart disease, and appears to help the immune system fight infection.

Iron protects against anemia; calcium helps build strong bones and protects against osteoporosis.

Navy Beans

FACTS Also known as great northern beans, haricot beans, or white kidney beans, at any name, this legume is worthy of recognition. Navy beans are very high in fiber—½ cup contains about 6 grams of dietary fiber. Navy beans are also a good source of potassium, iron, B vitamins, and other minerals.

Navy beans—the beans in Boston baked beans—are so named because at one time, they were a fixture in the Navy mess. Today, they are commonly used in soups and casseroles.

Beans are good for just about everyone, but they are especially beneficial for diabetics. Researchers at the University of Kentucky found that diabetics can lower their fasting blood sugar levels and reduce their cholesterol by adding 8 ounces of beans to their daily diet. Beans are complex carbohydrates, that is, it takes the body a lot longer to break down their molecules into simple sugars than, for example, sweets, which are high in sugar and are quickly metabolized. As a result, the body digests beans slowly, avoiding a sudden jump in glucose (blood sugar) levels that is dangerous to diabetics.

POSSIBLE BENEFITS   Beans contain soluble and insoluble fiber. Soluble fiber helps to reduce blood cholesterol levels, which cuts the risk of heart disease, diabetes, and stroke.

Insoluble fiber helps to promote bowel regularity, and is believed to reduce the risk of colon and rectal cancer.

Beans are low in fat: a diet low in fat reduces your risk of developing heart disease and certain forms of cancer.

Oat Bran

FACTS   Long before cholesterol became a household word—back in the days when heart disease was a relatively rare affliction—many Americans began the day with a heaping bowl of oatmeal. By the middle of the twentieth century, however, oatmeal was replaced in many households by higher-fat fare such as bacon and eggs and pancakes drenched in butter and imitation syrup. But in the 1980s, when "cholesterol fever" swept the country, oatmeal made a strong comeback after several leading medical journals reported that oat bran, which is rich in soluble fiber, could reduce cholesterol by as much as 12 percent. Suddenly, people were scarfing down Cheerios by the carton, and oat bran was being added to everything from muffins to brownies as food manufacturers tried to cash in on the public fear of heart disease. In 1990, however, oat bran fell into disrepute after a single study in the *Journal of the American Medical Association* concluded that oat bran was no more effective than white bread in lowering cholesterol. Almost overnight, oat bran became as passé as the Pet Rock.

Well, here's good news for oat bran lovers: Recent studies have vindicated this grain. Although it may not be a panacea, it does help reduce cholesterol and it does work better than white bread. Here's the evidence. Researchers from the University of Minnesota carefully scrutinized 10 studies on oat bran. They discovered that, on average, eating 3 grams of oat bran a day (roughly the amount in three packets of instant oatmeal) can result in a reduction of total cholesterol by 5–6 points. Although this doesn't sound very dramatic, this slight decrease in cholesterol can reduce your risk of heart disease by as much as 12 percent.

Oat bran appears to be even more effective for people with high cholesterol. For example, a recent study at the University of Kentucky College of Medicine, well known for its research on fiber, put 20 high cholesterol men on a diet high in oat bran. On average, the men had a 12.8 percent decline in total cholesterol and, even better, a 12.1 percent decline in LDL or "bad" cholesterol. When the same group of men were fed wheat bran, there was virtually no change in cholesterol. There's a valuable lesson to be learned from the oat bran saga. The rules of good nutrition don't change overnight; the results of a single study should not alter our eating habits.

Like other cereal grains, oat bran contains cancer-fighting compounds called phytates.

POSSIBLE BENEFITS Helps to reduce serum cholesterol levels, thus reducing the risk of coronary artery disease and stroke.

Phytates deactivate potent hormones that can trigger the growth of tumors.

PERSONAL ADVICE If you want to add oat bran, or any other form of fiber to your diet, do so slowly. Give your body time to adjust. Too much too soon could result in gas and indigestion.

If you have high cholesterol, you may want to talk to your physician about using oat bran. A high oat bran diet, along with other forms of soluble fiber, may be a more palatable treatment than some of the cholesterol-lowering drugs, which have some very unpleasant side effects.

Okra

FACTS If you're familiar with New Orleans cooking, you have undoubtedly eaten okra. The gluey sap from the pods is used to thicken a Cajun stew called gumbo. Okra is a superstar in terms of dietary fiber: ½ cup of cooked okra has almost 4 grams of fiber, which makes it one of the best vegetable sources around. Although it is not a superstar in terms of vitamins, it plays a significant supporting role. A ½ cup serving of okra provides about 10 percent of the RDA for beta-carotene, 20 percent of the day's supply of vitamin C, and a good amount of potassium.

POSSIBLE BENEFITS A high-fiber diet may help to prevent various forms of cancer, including colon/rectal. Some forms of fiber also reduce cholesterol.

Beta-carotene (the plant form of vitamin A) and vitamin C are both antioxidants which may help prevent the kind of cellular mutations that are prone to cancerous growth. Antioxidants also help to prevent the formation of plaque in vital arteries that can lead to heart attack and stroke.

Olive Oil

FACTS For years, scientists have been puzzled by the fact that the rate of heart disease was significantly lower in Mediterranean countries, like Greece, Italy, Spain, and southern France, yet the average intake of fat and cholesterol in those countries was similar to that in the United States. In fact, the Greek island of Crete consumes more olive oil than anywhere else on earth! Yet, their incidence of heart disease is minuscule compared with North America. To find out what was protecting Mediterranean people against heart disease, researchers took a closer look at the Mediterranean diet. Unlike the typical Western diet, which is high in saturated fat, the Mediterranean diet is high in monounsaturated fat, mainly in the form of olive oil. Numerous studies have shown that olive oil has a very special effect on blood cholesterol levels; although olive oil may not reduce total cholesterol, it does increase the amount of HDL or "good" cholesterol. High HDL levels are associated with lower rates of heart disease. Olive oil is not the only good thing about the Mediterranean diet—it is also high in complex carbohydrates and fiber. However, olive oil may be a contributing factor in protecting people against the ravages of heart disease.

At this point, scientists are not exactly sure how olive oil raises HDL; however, there are some interesting studies that may shed some light on this question. Recently, Israeli scientists studied the effect of olive oil on blood lipids as compared with a polyunsaturated oil. The researchers discovered that olive oil was less prone to oxidative damage than the polyunsaturated oil. This result is very interesting, considering the fact that oxidative damage of blood lipids is believed to be a major risk factor for developing atherosclerosis. Although there is still a great deal to be learned about olive oil, I feel we know enough about its beneficial effects to make it an everyday part of our lives.

POSSIBLE BENEFITS Helps prevent coronary artery disease by increasing HDL or "good" cholesterol.

PERSONAL ADVICE As good as olive oil may be, it is still a fat and should be ingested in limited quantities. Don't add olive oil to your diet without eliminating another form of fat. Stick to 1 or 2 tablespoons a day sprinkled on your salad, or use it in cooking instead of butter or polyunsaturated fat. Extra virgin olive oil has the best flavor and texture.

Onion

FACTS Onion is one of the 500 plants belonging to the genus *Allium,* which includes other illustrious members such as garlic, chives, and leek. For thousands of years, onion has been used in cooking, as well as by healers to treat a variety of ailments ranging from colds to athlete's foot.

Today, onion is high up on the list of foods being investigated by the National Cancer Institute for its potential cancer-fighting properties.

Onion attracted the attention of serious researchers in 1989 when the *Journal of the National Cancer Institute* published a Chinese study that noted that people who ate the highest amounts of allium vegetables had the lowest rates of stomach cancer. Several other studies have shown that various chemicals in onions can inhibit the growth of cancerous cells in animals and in test tube experiments.

The chemistry of the onion is very complex and has baffled chemists for nearly a century: it has more than 100 sulfur-containing compounds, many extremely exotic and complicated structures. It also is rich in flavonoids, including quercetin, which has been widely studied because it has been shown to deactivate several potent carcinogens and tumor promoters. According to a review article on quercetin by University of California, Berkeley, researcher Terrance Leighton, Ph.D., and colleagues, quercetin also interferes with the growth of estrogen-sensitive cells, the kinds of cells that are often involved in breast cancer. (Red and yellow onions and shallots have the highest flavonoid content of allium vegetables.)

Eric Block, Ph.D., of the State University of New York, Albany, recently discovered a sulfur compound in onion that in test tube studies can prevent the biochemical chain of events that lead to asthma and inflammatory reactions. Interestingly enough, onion has been used as a traditional remedy for respiratory ailments.

Onion appears to have a positive effect on cholesterol. Studies show that people who eat an onion a day can raise their HDL or "good" cholesterol. This vegetable may also help to lower blood pressure and prevent blood clots.

POSSIBLE BENEFITS May offer protection against cancer by inhibiting the growth of malignant tumors.

May help to prevent the inflammatory response that can lead to allergies and asthma.

May help to prevent heart attack and stroke by lowering cholesterol and blood pressure and preventing blood clots.

PERSONAL ADVICE A sprig of parsley can help clear the air of "onion breath," or look for an internal breath freshener made from parsley seed oil.

Orange

FACTS When you think of oranges you think of vitamin C, for good reason. One medium-size orange contains 70 mg of ascorbic acid, which is 10 mg more than the RDA for nonsmoking adults. It also offers a respectable 270 mg of potassium, 2.4 grams of fiber, and 270 IU of beta-carotene.

The National Cancer Institute is investigating this member of the citrus family because it contains many important chemically active substances that have been shown, at least in animal models, to help prevent cancer. For example, limonene, a citrus oil, has been shown to shrink mammary tumors in rats and prevent the growth of new tumors. The NCI is currently studying whether limonene and other citrus oils will have the same positive affect on humans. Other chemicals of interest in oranges include:

- Flavonoids—some are antioxidants—protect cells from damage by free radicals. Others may prevent the spread of malignant cells.

♦ Terpenes limit the production of cholesterol and help produce enzymes that deactivate carcinogens.

Most Americans don't eat the whole orange, they drink the juice. Freshly squeezed orange juice is a good choice. One cup of orange juice contains 124 mg of vitamin C, 500 mg of beta-carotene, and 496 mg of potassium. However, it does not have the fiber content of the whole orange. Therefore, I believe that drinking OJ is no substitute for the real thing.

POSSIBLE BENEFITS Vitamin C helps protect against many forms of cancer, including cervical, pancreatic, rectal, bladder, lung, and breast cancer.

Vitamin C helps fight heart disease by preventing the oxidation of LDL or "bad" cholesterol, which can lead to the formation of plaque in vital arteries.

Vitamin C can lessen the intensity of colds.

Vitamin C can help prevent infertility in men by preventing damage to the DNA in sperm.

The fiber in an orange can help maintain bowel regularity and lower cholesterol.

People with high levels of serum vitamin C have lower blood pressure than those with low levels of C.

Potassium helps to maintain normal fluid and electrolyte balance in the cells, as well as normal heart function and blood pressure.

PERSONAL ADVICE When you are buying OJ, look for the words "not from concentrate" on the label. OJ made from concentrate is too high in sugar.

Orange Roughy

FACTS Because it is less expensive than some of the more well-known fish, such as salmon and bass, orange roughy is beginning to appear on more and more restaurant menus. Native to New Zealand, this fish is usually sold frozen in fillets and steaks. It has a very mild flavor, which makes it a good choice for people who contend that they hate anything remotely "fishy." It is also a dieter's dream: one 4-ounce serving contains a scant 100 calories and virtually no saturated fat.

POSSIBLE BENEFITS Extremely low in fat, orange roughy can help reduce the risk of developing coronary artery disease and certain forms of cancer.

PERSONAL ADVICE Orange roughy is a good choice for people worried about contaminants in fish. First, since toxins are stored in fatty tissue, a fat-free fish will retain fewer contaminants than a fatty one. Second, it comes from waters that are relatively clean.

Oysters

FACTS For centuries, oysters have had a reputation for being an aphrodisiac—it's not as farfetched as it sounds. Oysters are extremely rich in zinc, a mineral that is essential for sperm formation and male potency. Oysters are also high in iron—one cup of raw oysters provides 15.6 mg of iron, slightly more than the RDA for men and women (pregnant women need 30 mg). To round out the nutritional picture, oysters are also a good source of vitamins A, B_{12}, and C. As seafood goes, oysters are high in cholesterol—one cup has about 120 mg of cholesterol, more than twice the amount in other fish. However, considering that it is a virtual reservoir of zinc, an occasional meal of oysters is probably worth it.

POSSIBLE BENEFITS Zinc has been used to treat impotency and infertility in men and is reputed to enhance the male sex drive.

Zinc is essential for normal taste, smell, and sight and for normal wound healing.

Recent studies show that zinc may be an immune booster and may prove to be as useful against the common cold as vitamin C.

Iron is necessary for the production of hemoglobin and certain enzymes.

PERSONAL ADVICE Never eat raw oysters. Steam them until they are thoroughly cooked.

Papaya

FACTS What's the best fruit to help you beat the common cold? If you guessed orange, you're wrong. Papaya has lots more vitamin C, which may not prevent colds, but can help lessen the severity of one. The numbers are very impressive: one papaya provides more than 300 percent of the RDA for vitamin C. In addition, it has more than a day's supply of beta-carotene (which is roughly five times the beta-carotene content of an orange). Papaya is also an excellent source of fiber and potassium.

Papaya juice is a traditional remedy for indigestion. Papaya contains a substance called papain which is similar to pepsin, an enzyme that helps digest protein in the body. Although scientists claim that the papain in papaya has no effect on digestion, I know many people who swear that papaya juice works better than over-the-counter antacids.

POSSIBLE BENEFITS Vitamin C helps the body to resist infection. An antioxidant, vitamin C is also believed to help prevent the formation of cancerous tumors, and may play a role in preventing atherosclerosis or hardening of the arteries.

Vitamin C may help boost fertility in men by preventing damage to sperm DNA.

Beta-carotene, also an antioxidant, may help to prevent many different forms of cancer. Beta-carotene may also help prevent oxidation of lipids that may contribute to the formation of plaque deposits in the arteries.

Potassium is essential for normal heart function and blood pressure.

Fiber helps to maintain bowel regularity and may help to prevent colon/rectal cancers.

Parsley

FACTS A cookbook written in the thirteenth century advises using parsley sprigs to decorate and add flavor to a variety of "meates both boyled and roasted." To this day, most of us think of this herb as a little more than a garnish. This is an unfortunate perception. Parsley is packed with vitamin C and beta-carotene and lots of other good things (10 sprigs provide 10 percent of the RDA for beta-carotene and 15 percent of the C).

Parsley is a member of the illustrious umbelliferous vegetable family, which is being investigated by the National Cancer Institute because of its cancer-fighting potential. Some of the biologically active substances in parsley include:

- Polyacetylenes, which block the synthesis of prostaglandins that may promote cancer
- Coumarins, which help prevent blood clotting and are also believed to have anticancer properties
- Flavonoids, some which work as antioxidants, others deactivating hormones that can trigger tumor growth
- Monoterpenes, antioxidants that help fight cancer and reduce cholesterol

POSSIBLE BENEFITS Beta-carotene may help protect against many different forms of cancer and heart disease.

Vitamin C protects against cancer and heart disease and helps strengthen the immune system.

The biologically active substances in parsley help prevent cancer and heart disease.

PERSONAL ADVICE On top of everything else, parsley is also a terrific breath freshener, and can help tame even the most difficult odors. So if you're following my advice and eating lots of garlic and onions, keep a few sprigs of parsley on hand at all times.

For a good-tasting tea that is chock full of beta-carotene, put 10 sprigs of parsley in a teapot. Pour hot water over the parsley and let steep for 10 minutes. Flavor with a little honey or lemon. This one is great for colds!

Parsnip

FACTS Parsnip is a member of the Umbelliferae family (along with carrots and celery) which is being investigated by the National Cancer Institute for its potential cancer-fighting properties. Parsnip looks like a washed-out carrot, but has its own distinctive flavor. Umbelliferous vegetables such as parsnip contain many important phytochemicals which, in laboratory and animal studies, have been shown to thwart the spread of cancerous cells. For example, terpenes, compounds common to Umbelliferae, appear to deactivate steroidal hormones that can promote the growth of certain types of tumors. Members of the Umbelliferae family also have polyacetylenes and phenolic acids, which have anti-inflammatory properties, and flavonoids, some of which deactivate carcinogens before they can alter a cell making it susceptible to cancerous growth.

Until the NCI has completed its research, we can't be certain that parsnip is a cancer fighter, but it certainly appears to be a likely candidate. We do know for a fact that this vegetable is a leader in dietary fiber—a ½ cup serving of cooked parsnip provides an impressive 3.3 grams of fiber, more than many so-called high-fiber breakfast cereals.

POSSIBLE BENEFITS May possess many important chemical compounds which prevent the initiation and growth of cancer cells.

Fiber helps to maintain bowel regularity and protects against colon and rectal cancer.

Peach

FACTS Here's a recipe for success. Take 2 grams of dietary fiber, 470 IU of beta-carotene (almost 10 percent of the RDA), a touch of potassium, and give it a delicious, sweet taste. Do it all for a mere 35 calories and zero fat. What you've got is a peach, which makes a terrific snack or dessert. With these numbers, why stop at just one?

POSSIBLE BENEFITS Beta-carotene, the plant form of vitamin A, is believed to protect against many different forms of cancer and heart disease.

Fiber is essential for normal digestion and may help to prevent colon/rectal cancer.

Low-calorie, low-fat foods help prevent obesity, a leading cause of heart disease, diabetes, and cancer.

Pear

FACTS If constipation is a chronic problem, you need to eat more foods like pear. One pear contains roughly 3 grams of dietary fiber—mostly insoluble fiber—which means that it promotes bowel regularity. One pear also contains 10 percent of the RDA for vitamin C, and a good amount of potassium. Pears are low in calories and fat, and very sweet, which makes them the perfect food for people with a sweet tooth who are watching their weight.

POSSIBLE BENEFITS Insoluble fiber can help prevent constipation and digestive disorders such as diverticulosis. It also can help prevent colon/rectal cancer.

Peas (Green)

FACTS If you were one of the countless children who used to pick the peas out of your peas and carrots, it's time to give this vegetable another try. Peas are packed with the kinds of vitamins and nutrients that can keep you healthy. A ½ cup serving of fresh, cooked peas contains more than 20 percent of the RDA for vitamin C, 10 percent of a day's supply of beta-carotene, and 8 percent of the RDA for iron. Peas are also a terrific source of fiber (2.5 grams per ½ cup) and potassium, which helps keep all of your body cells functioning properly.

POSSIBLE BENEFITS Vitamin C helps improve your resistance against infection, and is also believed to help prevent certain forms of cancer.

Beta-carotene, the plant form of vitamin A, may protect against various forms of cancer and heart disease.

Potassium is essential for normal heart function and can lower blood pressure.

Fiber, which most Americans do not get enough of, can help prevent colon/rectal cancer and can reduce cholesterol.

Peppers (Red)

FACTS Sweet red peppers may not be as "hot" these days as the trendier chili peppers, but in terms of good nutrition, they have a sizzle all of their own. One pepper provides more than 150 percent of the RDA for vitamin C for non-smokers—in fact, it is one of nature's best sources of this vitamin (oranges don't even come close).

The average red pepper has 4220 IU of beta-carotene, more than 80 percent of the RDA for this vitamin.

Red pepper is also one of the few foods to contain lycopene, a carotenoid that may help to prevent various forms of cancer. Recent studies show that people with low levels of lycopene are at greater risk of developing cancers of the cervix, bladder, and pancreas.

POSSIBLE BENEFITS Beta-carotene may help to prevent coronary artery disease.

Carotenoids (such as lycopene) may help to prevent many different types of cancer.

Beta-carotene may help prevent the cellular damage that leads to premature aging.

Popcorn

FACTS When you begin to trim your diet of excess calories and fat, very often the snack foods are the first to go. Potato chips, processed cheese snacks, corn chips, and the like are packed with fat and calories, and little else. Well, take comfort in knowing that there is still one "fun food" that is good enough for the Hot Hundred—popcorn. The new "lite" versions of this popular snack food, lower in fat and sodium than the old-fashioned kind, are actually good for you. Depending on the brand, a 3-cup serving of popcorn provides roughly 3 grams of dietary fiber, between 3 and 4 grams of fat, and fewer than 100 calories. Compare this with a mere 1 ounce of potato chips which weighs in at 150 calories, 10 grams of fat, and very little fiber (not to mention the fact that very few people can stop at 1 ounce). When you feel a need to snack, popcorn is your best choice.

POSSIBLE BENEFITS Will soothe your craving for a snack food, but will not load you up with fat and calories.

PERSONAL ADVICE To reduce fat, I make popcorn in a hot-air popper (a low-fat, low-sodium, microwave popcorn is also a good choice). I add a small amount of corn oil, or another lightly flavored monounsaturated or polyunsaturated vegetable oil, to prevent sticking. When cooked, sprinkle on a low-sodium herbal seasoning. If you can eat yeast, add a little nutritional yeast for flavor and a touch of B-complex vitamins. This popcorn tastes delicious, and is terrific for you. If you need a buttery taste, try one of the commercial powdered butter-flavored products or add a little corn oil.

Pork Loin

FACTS Pork has become synonymous with fat; yet, many cuts of pork are relatively lean and, calorie for calorie, are an excellent source of vitamins and minerals. For example, a well-trimmed broiled loin chop is 165 calories and 8 grams of fat, not bad considering that 3 ounces of rib roast has 26 fat grams, or 3 ounces of leg of lamb has 13 fat grams. Pork is also an excellent source of vitamin A and iron, and a reasonably good source of B vitamins, zinc, and folic acid.

POSSIBLE BENEFITS Can provide vitamins and minerals that are essential for good body functioning.

Pregnant women take note: pork is rich in folic acid, which can help prevent birth defects.

Vitamin B_6 and zinc help boost the immune system.

PERSONAL ADVICE When it comes to meat, watch your portion size.

Potato (White)

FACTS The poor, much maligned potato! When the dieting craze began in the late 1960s, potatoes fell out of favor because they were mistakenly labeled "fattening." It always amazed me how people would gobble up a pound of steak, fat and all, and then push the baked potato to the side because they were "watching their weight." Knowledgeable weight watchers, however, know that the potato is a dieter's dream. At 220 calories per potato and virtually no fat, it can make a filling and satisfying meal. It is also loaded with good things. It contains 26 mg of vitamin C, nearly half of the RDA for nonsmokers. It also has an impressive 844 mg of potassium, nearly twice as much as is in a banana! White potatoes are also a good source of vitamin B_6 and, to a lesser extent, the other B vitamins, and an excellent source of fiber (4.1 grams).

POSSIBLE BENEFITS Vitamin C is good for so many things—it protects against cancer and heart disease as well as helps boost the immune system.

Potassium is essential to maintain fluid and electrolyte balance in the cells, as well as normal heart function and blood pressure.

Vitamin B_6 helps strengthen the immune system.

Fiber helps to maintain bowel regularity and protect against rectal and colon cancers.

CAUTION Do not eat the potato skin, which is typically sprayed with a sprout inhibitor that may prove to be toxic. Peel your potatoes before cooking or eat around the skin.

PERSONAL ADVICE Don't ruin a perfectly good baked potato by loading it up with high-fat garnishes such as butter, margarine, or sour cream. Instead use olive oil or powdered nonfat butter flavoring, or plain no-fat yogurt flavored with chives.

Potato juice is a wonderful antacid. In Germany, it is a common remedy for indigestion. To make potato juice, peel two potatoes and put them in a juicer.

Prune

FACTS Prunes are a well-known cure for constipation, but they also perform some other important tasks. Researchers at the University of California at Davis and the University of Minnesota investigated whether prunes, an excellent source of soluble fiber, could lower cholesterol. The eight-week study was divided into two parts: During the first part, 41 men with mildly elevated blood cholesterol levels were given 350 ml of grape juice daily in addition to their normal diet. During the second half, the same men were taken off grape juice and given 12 prunes a day (6 grams dietary fiber). The results: During the prune period, the total cholesterol levels dipped slightly, but more important, the LDL or "bad" cholesterol dropped dramatically as compared with the grape juice part of the study.

The researchers also examined whether prunes had any effect on concentrations of fecal bile acid—this is important because high levels of certain acids are associated with an increased risk of colon cancer. One particular acid, lithocholic acid, was lower after the prune period than after the grape juice period, which suggests that prunes may offer some protection against colon cancer.

Prunes are also a good source of beta-carotene—five large

prunes have 970 IU of beta-carotene, nearly a fifth of the RDA. Prunes are also a good source of copper and boron.

POSSIBLE BENEFITS By reducing LDL cholesterol, prunes may reduce the risk of coronary artery disease and stroke.

By promoting bowel regularity and reducing the concentration of lithocholic acid, prunes may help prevent colon cancer.

Beta-carotene also helps protect against various forms of cancer and heart disease.

Copper may help to prevent blood clots.

Boron appears to help postmenopausal women retain estrogen, which is necessary for calcium absorption.

PERSONAL ADVICE If you want to add prunes to your diet, do so slowly to avoid any gas or discomfort. Remember that five large prunes weigh in at about 115 calories, so if you're watching your weight, you need to eliminate roughly the same amount of calories from other food sources to make room for prunes.

Psyllium

FACTS Derived from the husks of psyllium seeds, this gel-forming soluble fiber is used in many bulk laxatives (for example, Metamucil) to promote bowel regularity and is also added to some ready-to-eat cereals. Psyllium has become "hot" in recent years because of its ability to lower cholesterol. For example, fiber expert James W. Anderson and others at the University of Kentucky Medical Service studied the effect of a diet rich in psyllium flake cereal or wheat bran flake cereal on the cholesterol levels of 44 people with high cholesterol. After six weeks, the average serum cholesterol levels of the psyllium group decreased by 12 percent, but the wheat bran group remained roughly the same. The so-called bad or LDL cholesterol decreased significantly among the psyllium group, but not among the wheat group.

POSSIBLE BENEFITS By lowering total cholesterol and LDLs, may reduce the risk of coronary artery disease and stroke.

By promoting bowel regularity, may reduce the risk of rectal and colon cancer.

CAUTION Psyllium can cause an allergic reaction in sensitive individuals. If you are allergic to many different foods, check with your allergist before trying psyllium. If you experience any allergic reaction after ingesting this food, call your physician immediately.

PERSONAL ADVICE Psyllium in bulk, without any added sugar or other sweeteners, can be purchased in natural foods stores.

Pumpkin

FACTS Most of the fresh pumpkins sold in the United States are carved into jack-o'-lanterns for Halloween, which is really a shame. Pumpkin, a variety of winter squash, is not only delicious, but is packed with good nutrition. Pumpkin is a terrific source of beta-carotene, as well as other vitamins and minerals. A ½ cup serving provides 25 percent of the RDA for beta-carotene, 10 percent of the RDA for vitamin

C, and a generous dose of potassium. It's also a good source of dietary fiber.

Although fresh pumpkin has a unique flavor and texture, canned pumpkin—the kind you use in pumpkin pie—is no less nutritious. In fact, ½ cup of pumpkin pie mix provides 220 percent of the RDA for beta-carotene and is fairly low in calories. Don't wait for Thanksgiving, this is a dessert you can eat all year round!

POSSIBLE BENEFITS Beta-carotene may help to prevent many different forms of cancer. It can also slightly reduce the risk of lung cancer for smokers.

Beta-carotene may help prevent atherosclerosis, or hardening of the arteries, which can lead to heart attack and stroke.

Vitamin C, a potent antioxidant, may protect against cancer and heart disease, and help the body fight against infection.

PERSONAL ADVICE There are three varieties of pumpkin that are good for cooking: sweet, sugar, or cheese pumpkins. Bake them in the oven like any other squash.

Pumpkin seed oil is a wonderful source of zinc and unsaturated fatty acids that can help against prostate problems. Dried and roasted pumpkin seeds are a source of this oil; however, more potent supplements are available in capsule form in natural food stores.

Quinoa

FACTS Quinoa (pronounced "keen-wa") has been touted as the "super grain of the future," but in reality, this food has been around for hundreds of years. Although it looks, cooks, and tastes like a grain, quinoa is not a grain at all— it's actually the dried fruit of an herb that is native to Bolivia and Peru. The Incas thought so highly of quinoa that they called it the "mother grain."

Quinoa is now being grown in the Rocky Mountains of Colorado, which has a climate and terrain similar to the Andes. Unlike traditional grains, quinoa is rich in all eight essential amino acids that compose a "complete protein," and are normally found only in red meat, eggs, and dairy products. However, quinoa has a decided edge over these other foods in that it is much lower in calories and fat and is abundant in fiber. One serving of quinoa (about ½ cup) has 129 calories, 2 grams of fat, and 4.6 grams of dietary fiber. Quinoa is also an excellent source of potassium and iron, and a good source of zinc and various B vitamins.

Until recently, quinoa was sold only in natural food stores, but today you can buy it packaged at the supermarket. It cooks in about 10–15 minutes, and has a mild flavor.

POSSIBLE BENEFITS   Quinoa provides high-quality protein that is normally found in meat.

Fiber can help prevent many digestive disorders as well as many different forms of cancer.

Potassium helps regulate blood pressure and heart function, which helps to prevent heart disease and stroke.

Zinc promotes healing of wounds and is also an immune booster.

Iron can help prevent anemia.

Raspberries

FACTS People who are watching their weight often feel that if a food is sweet and delicious, it can't possibly be allowed on their diet. Raspberries prove them wrong. This fruit is bursting with flavor, but not with calories or fat. A 1-cup serving of raspberries is a mere 100 calories. However, it contains about half the RDA for vitamin C, an impressive 3.3 grams of dietary fiber, and a fair amount of potassium. If you feel a "dessert attack" coming on, try eating a cup of fresh raspberries—for a real treat, top it off with a dollop of low-fat whipped "cream" made from evaporated skim milk. I guarantee that your urge to binge will disappear.

POSSIBLE BENEFITS Raspberries can help you stick to a low-fat diet without feeling deprived.

Fiber helps to promote bowel regularity and may protect against various forms of cancer.

Vitamin C protects against cancer and cardiovascular disease and is an immune booster.

Potassium helps to prevent stroke and heart attack by normalizing blood pressure.

Red Kidney Beans

FACTS Best known for their starring role in chili, these good-tasting beans are simply packed with fiber: ½ cup serving contains a whopping 7.3 grams of dietary fiber. Red kidney beans are an excellent source of potassium and folic acid, and a good source of iron.

Vegetarians take note: these beans are also a good plant

source of protein. However, they contain only a few of the eight essential amino acids that the body needs but cannot produce itself. Therefore, they need to be teamed up with a complementing food, such as rice, to create a complete protein.

Eating any kind of bean—but especially one that is as high in fiber as red kidney beans—can have a wonderful effect on your cholesterol level. According to studies done at the University of Kentucky, well known for its research on dietary fiber, eating at least 4 ounces of cooked beans daily can reduce cholesterol levels of over 200 mg/dl by as much as 20 percent.

POSSIBLE BENEFITS Fiber helps speed the passage of food through the GI tract, which not only promotes bowel regularity but may protect against colon cancer.

By cutting blood cholesterol levels, red kidney beans can help reduce the risk of diabetes, stroke, and cardiovascular disease.

Folic acid helps protect against neural tube defects developing in the fetus, various forms of cancer, and heart disease.

Potassium helps to maintain normal blood pressure which can help prevent heart attack and stroke.

PERSONAL ADVICE In some individuals, bean consumption leads to a gaseous digestive tract. Antigas products that break down the gas-causing substances in beans are now readily available in supermarkets, drugstores, and natural food stores. However, people who are allergic to mold should avoid these products.

Red Snapper

`FACTS` This fish has a unique, delicate flavor that distinguishes it from the others. It is also extremely low in calories and fat. A 3½-ounce serving is a scant 100 calories, with only 1.34 grams of fat and 37 mg of cholesterol. Red snapper tastes so good that you won't want to smother its natural flavor in a heavy sauce, which makes it an excellent food for "waist watchers."

`POSSIBLE BENEFITS` A low-fat diet can help reduce the risk of heart disease and certain forms of cancer.

Rhubarb

`FACTS` It doesn't come from an animal that moos, nor is it white and creamy, yet this remarkable fruit is chock full of calcium. One cup of cooked rhubarb has a whopping 348 mg of calcium, more than a cup of milk, but without a trace of the fat. One cup of cooked rhubarb will provide men and premenopausal women with a third of their daily requirement of calcium. It provides one fifth of the calcium RDA for postmenopausal women.

The problem is, rhubarb is not exactly common fare. In fact, other than an occasional piece of rhubarb pie, few people take advantage of this terrific fruit. It's not hard to find—you've probably walked by it hundreds of times at the produce section of your supermarket. Rhubarb resembles celery, except it has larger leaves and a thicker, pink stem. The stem can be chopped and boiled in water. Naturally bitter, rhubarb needs to be sweetened with honey, or combined with a sweet fruit like strawberry.

POSSIBLE BENEFITS   The calcium in rhubarb is essential for strong teeth and bones and helps prevent osteoporosis; helps maintain normal blood pressure and heart function; protects against certain forms of cancer, including rectal cancer.

PERSONAL ADVICE   Only the stem is edible: Do not eat the leaves of the rhubarb plant. They contain oxalic acid, which is toxic.

Rhubarb is a terrific alternative source of calcium for people who are lactose-intolerant—it should be a regular part of their diet. However, to maintain rhubarb's healthy advantage, try to cook it with as little sweetener as possible, and don't douse it with fat—a small amount will do.

Rosemary

FACTS   As more and more people begin to reduce their sodium intake, undoubtedly herbs such as rosemary will be rediscovered. Sprigs of fresh rosemary leaves can enhance the flavor of most meats, fish, and salads. However, rosemary has earned a slot in the Hot Hundred not because of its delicate flavor, but because of its cancer-fighting potential. Rosemary contains chemicals called quinones, which in laboratory studies have been shown to inhibit carcinogens and cocarcinogens (chemicals that enhance the action of cancer-causing substances).

Rosemary is an ancient folk remedy for improving memory. It's also been used by herbalists to treat dizziness due to inner ear disturbances.

POSSIBLE BENEFITS   Rosemary may deactivate carcinogens, and thus prevent the initiation and spread of cancer.

Salmon

FACTS   Popular but pricey, salmon has come into its own as people are becoming more aware of the heart-healthy benefits of eating fish. There are several kinds of salmon: Red or sockeye salmon is the kind that is typically sold in cans. Coho or Atlantic salmon is sold in posh restaurants or at fish stores. Although any kind of salmon offers a fair amount of fatty fish oil, Atlantic salmon is fin and gill above the rest—one 4-ounce serving has a whopping 2.1 grams of omega-3 fatty acids, making it one of the best natural sources of omega-3. Canned salmon with bone is also an excellent source of calcium, providing 20 percent of the RDA, as well as vitamin D, which is essential for the absorption of this important mineral. All species of salmon are low in calories and cholesterol unless doused in butter or suffocated by a fattening sauce.

POSSIBLE BENEFITS   Omega-3 fatty acids:

+ May lower cholesterol and triglycerides in people with elevated blood lipids, thus reducing their risk of coronary artery disease
+ May help retard the growth of cancerous tumors
+ May prevent dangerous blood clots that can lead to heart attack and stroke

♦ May help reduce inflammation caused by conditions such as psoriasis, arthritis, and lupus
♦ Calcium is essential for building strong bones and for normal heart function and blood pressure

PERSONAL ADVICE   Baked, poached, or broiled is the way I like my salmon. Try putting it in salads, or in a salmon club sandwich on whole grain bread.

Sardines

FACTS   Sardines canned in oil are a good source of omega-3 fatty acids (0.7 gram per 4-ounce serving). Although they are somewhat higher in calories than many other fish—236 calories per 4-ounce serving—they offer a few things that other fish don't. For one thing, sardine bones are a good source of calcium, providing 10 percent of the RDA. For another, they are rich in nucleic acids, RNA and DNA, substances that some researchers believe may retard the aging process. Here's how. The body is made up of millions of cells, the average cell having a life span of roughly two years. Before a cell dies, it reproduces itself, but with each reproduction, it goes through some changes, not necessarily for the better. In other words, it begins to wear out. Nucleic acids may help produce healthier cells that are able to live longer, thus retarding the aging process.

POSSIBLE BENEFITS   Omega-3 fatty acids:

♦ May lower cholesterol in people with elevated cholesterol and reduce triglycerides
♦ May help to prevent the growth of cancerous tumors

♦ May help to prevent blood clots, thus reducing the risk of heart attack and stroke
♦ Are essential for normal brain and eye development

Calcium helps to build strong bones and to maintain normal blood pressure and heart function.

Nucleic acids may help you live longer and look younger.

PERSONAL ADVICE Water-packed sardines are available for those who want less oil and fat in their diet.

Shiitake and Reishi Mushrooms

FACTS Thrown into soup or pasta, or sautéed by themselves in a little olive oil, these Asian mushrooms are popping up at some of the best restaurants in town. They are quite expensive, but may be worth their weight in gold. Although there are some differences between reishi and shiitake, there are many similarities.

Both are potential cancer fighters. Recent studies show that extract from reishi mushroom can stop the growth of cancerous tumors in mice. Other studies suggest that reishi has antihistamine action that can help control allergies.

Several studies have shown that a compound of shiitake, lentinan, can stimulate the immune system to fight off viral infections and tumor cells. In fact, lentinan is used as a cancer treatment in Japan.

Even if these mushrooms turn out to be potent medicine, fortunately they do not taste the slightest bit medicinal. These mushrooms are absolutely delicious, and at 40 calories per one cup (cooked) are a true caloric bargain. Better yet, they are fat-free, sodium-free, and a good source of riboflavin and niacin (roughly one third of the RDA for each).

POSSIBLE BENEFITS   Reishi mushrooms may protect against cancer.

Lentinan from shiitake mushrooms may help boost the immune system and may also help the body fight off tumor cells.

Riboflavin helps the body release energy from food.

Niacin is essential for the metabolism of carbohydrates. A recent study suggests that low blood levels of niacin may promote cancer.

Spinach

FACTS   Popeye was right! "Eat your spinach" has been the rallying cry of mothers through the ages. We should have listened. This green, leafy vegetable has a lot to offer. It is rich in beta-carotene—one cup raw spinach has 3690 IU of beta-carotene, or roughly 70 percent of the RDA). It is also a good source of vitamin B_6, folic acid, iron, and potassium. Spinach also provides better than 10 percent of the RDA for riboflavin, vitamin C, calcium, and magnesium.

POSSIBLE BENEFITS   Beta-carotene may protect against developing various forms of cancer and heart disease.

Folic acid helps prevent birth defects, certain types of cancer, and heart disease.

Potassium helps maintain normal electrolyte balance within each cell and helps normalize heart function and blood pressure.

B_6 is good for the immune system; so is vitamin C.

Iron helps prevent iron-deficiency anemia.

Calcium and magnesium are good for many things, including building strong bones and normalizing blood pressure.

PERSONAL ADVICE Vitamin C helps absorb iron; therefore, adding lemon juice to your spinach is a good idea.

Strawberry

FACTS Freshly picked, ripe strawberries are one of nature's finest gifts—they're sweet, they taste terrific, and they're exceptionally low in calories. One cup of strawberries weighs in at a mere 45 calories, a pretty impressive figure that can help you maintain your figure. Strawberries are also very high in vitamin C—one cup provides 82 mg of vitamin C, 120 percent of the RDA. Not only that, strawberries are high in fiber, offering 2.2 grams per cup.

If all this wasn't enough to earn the strawberry a place in the food hall of fame, the fact that it contains ellagic acid makes it very special indeed. Only two other fruits—grapes and cherries—contain this special compound which has been shown to prevent carcinogens from turning healthy cells into cancerous ones.

POSSIBLE BENEFITS Vitamin C helps protect against various forms of cancer.

As an antioxidant, vitamin C helps prevent oxidation of LDL or "bad" cholesterol, which can lead to atherosclerosis.

Fiber helps maintain bowel regularity and protect against colon and rectal cancer.

Ellagic acid may help prevent cancer by deactivating carcinogens before they can do their dirty work.

Sweet Potato

FACTS How did Scarlett O'Hara keep her 19-inch waist-line? Her nanny used to force her to load up on sweet potatoes before going out to a party so that Scarlett wouldn't eat any of the more fattening party fare. Her nanny knew what she was doing. One sweet potato can make a significant dent in even the most voracious appetites, at a mere 115 calories and no fat.

Sweet potatoes also pack a significant nutritional wallop. Rich in beta-carotene, one medium-size potato contains five times the RDA for vitamin A (24,880 IU)! Sweet potato is also an excellent source of potassium (roughly one half the RDA).

POSSIBLE BENEFITS High levels of serum beta-carotene reduce the risk of developing various forms of cancer, including cancers of the breast, ovary, cervix, and bladder.

Beta-carotene also appears to protect against atherosclerosis, which can lead to heart attack and stroke.

Potassium helps maintain fluid and electrolyte balance in the body cells, as well as normal heart function and blood pressure.

Wild Mexican yams, which are related to sweet potato, seem to have antiweight-gain, anticancer and antiaging properties.

Tangerine

FACTS Tangerine may be the perfect snack food. It comes in its own convenient wrapper, and at 35 calories per fruit, it helps satisfy your sweet tooth without compromising your waistline. It is rich in antioxidants: one tangerine provides 45 percent of the RDA for vitamin C and 15 percent of beta-carotene. As a member of the illustrious citrus family—which is being studied by the National Cancer Institute—tangerine contains a number of disease-fighting phytochemicals, including flavonoids, which help protect against cancer, and terpenes, which limit the production of cholesterol.

POSSIBLE BENEFITS Vitamin C and beta-carotene help prevent heart disease and many different forms of cancer.

Vitamin C can lessen the severity and duration of the common cold.

Some flavonoids are antioxidants which help prevent cancer and premature aging. Others may halt the spread of malignant cells.

Terpenes help prevent coronary artery disease and produce enzymes that deactivate carcinogens.

Tofu (Bean Curd)

FACTS A staple of Oriental cuisine, tofu or bean curd is made from dry soybeans, which are soaked and then crushed and boiled. A coagulant is added to the liquid portion, or soy milk, to make it separate into curds and whey. The fresh, warm curds are poured into molds and left to settle. The result: the custardy, white tofu that is sold in greengroceries, supermarkets, and natural food stores. Tofu has a very mild, almost bland flavor that easily soaks up the flavors of other foods and spices. It can be used as a meat or cheese substitute in such dishes as chili or lasagna.

Tofu is high in protein, cholesterol-free, and low in calories. (Six ounces weighs in at 100 calories.) Tofu that is made with calcium sulfate is a good source of calcium, providing roughly a third of the RDA for this mineral.

Like any other soybean products, tofu is rich in isoflavones, compounds that are phytoestrogens, that is, hormone-like substances that mimic the action of estrogen in humans. Phytoestrogens may offer many of the beneficial effects of estrogen without any of the negative aspects. For example, Japanese women—who eat lots of tofu, bean sprouts, and other soy products—rarely complain of menopausal symptoms such as hot flashes, which are quite common among Western women. In fact, millions of Western women take synthetic estrogen replacement therapy to alleviate these symptoms. However, unlike synthetic estrogens, phytoestrogens do not increase the risk of developing certain forms of cancer. In fact, quite the opposite is true. Studies show that women who eat foods rich in soy isoflavones have lower rates of breast cancer than those who don't.

Isoflavones may also help men. Japanese men, who routinely eat a diet high in soy products, also have lower rates of prostate cancer than Western men.

Recently, a new compound called genistein was found in the urine of people who eat foods rich in soy. Genistein blocks the growth of new capillaries that supply blood to some tumors, thus denying the tumors their source of nutrients. As a result, genistein may help to prevent the spread of cancer.

POSSIBLE BENEFITS   The calcium in tofu helps strengthen bones and maintain normal heart function.

Calcium helps maintain normal blood pressure and may protect against certain forms of cancer.

Isoflavones may help protect against various forms of cancer.

Isoflavones may help reduce the discomfort of menopause.

PERSONAL ADVICE Tofu "ice cream" is a delicious alternative dessert for people with lactose intolerance. It also can be made into a terrific cheesecake.

Tomato

FACTS A tomato a day may be the difference between developing cancer and living cancer-free. Tomatoes are one of a handful of fruits and vegetables that are rich in a carotenoid called lycopene. Recent studies show that people who have the highest blood levels of lycopene are at much lower risk of developing various forms of cancer including cancers of the cervix, bladder, and pancreas. In order to achieve this protective level of lycopene, just eat one tomato a day. More good news—lycopene is also present in processed tomato products such as tomato juice and tomato paste.

Tomato is also an excellent source of vitamin C (22 mg or more than a third of the RDA for nonsmokers) and has 1 gram of fiber.

POSSIBLE BENEFITS Lycopene and vitamin C may help prevent various forms of cancer.

Vitamin C helps boost the immune system.

Fiber may help to prevent colon/rectal cancer.

PERSONAL ADVICE Rheumatoid arthritis sufferers note: the nightshades, such as potatoes, tomatoes, and eggplant, may aggravate this condition.

Trout

FACTS Trout is a good source of omega-3 fatty acids (1.1 grams per 4-ounce serving) and is low in saturated fat and calories. This fish is rich in vitamin B_{12} and provides more than 10 percent of the RDA for iron. Unfortunately, trout is found in lakes and streams, many of which have become dumping grounds for polluters. Therefore, try to buy trout that has been raised on a fish farm.

POSSIBLE BENEFITS Omega-3 fatty acids:

♦ May lower cholesterol and triglycerides, which can reduce your risk of developing coronary artery disease
♦ May lower blood pressure and prevent dangerous blood clots, which can help prevent heart attack and stroke
♦ May prevent the growth of cancerous tumors
♦ Are essential for normal brain and eye development

Iron and vitamin B_{12} can help prevent anemia. B_{12} deficiency in older people can cause memory loss, confusion, mood changes, and other neurological symptoms.

Tuna

FACTS Albacore white-meat tuna canned in water is an excellent low-calorie, low-cholesterol way to get a reasonably good dose of omega-3 fatty acids (0.8 mg per 4-ounce serving). It also has more than 40 percent of the RDA for vitamin B_{12} and is a good source of niacin.

Don't scrimp and buy the cheaper light tuna—you may be saving a few pennies, but you're losing a lot of the omega-3 fatty acids, which is why you're eating this fish in the first place.

If you make tuna salad, remember to hold the mayo. The heart-healthy benefits of tuna are quickly canceled out if you load it up with extra fat—regular mayo is up to 80 percent fat! Use lemon juice or low-fat salad dressing instead.

Fresh tuna is delicious but expensive. In many cases, it may not be as rich in omega-3 as the canned albacore tuna.

POSSIBLE BENEFITS Omega 3 fatty acids:

- May reduce high cholesterol levels and normalize elevated blood pressure, thus reducing the risk of heart disease and stroke
- May prevent the formation of dangerous blood clots
- May help retard the growth of cancerous tumors
- Are essential for normal brain and eye development

Vitamin B_{12} is necessary for the body to utilize folic acid and can help prevent anemia. This vitamin can also prevent neurological symptoms in older people that resemble Alzheimer's disease.

Niacin is essential for the metabolism of carbohydrates, and may offer some protection against cancer.

PERSONAL ADVICE Unfortunately, tuna is one of the fish that is contaminated by mercury. But albacore tuna, a deepwater fish, is usually less polluted. Nevertheless, most people can eat tuna safely; however, pregnant women should limit their intake to 7 ounces a week.

Turkey

FACTS   For some reason, Americans save turkey for special occasions like Thanksgiving and Christmas, but it's actually the kind of food that we should be eating all year round. Turkey is very low in fat—there's only 1 fat gram per ounce of flesh (minus the skin), and most of that fat is polyunsaturated. A 5-ounce serving of turkey is a mere 220 calories, but provides nearly 50 percent of the RDA for folic acid. It is also a moderately good source of vitamins B_1 and B_6, zinc, and potassium.

POSSIBLE BENEFITS   Eating turkey instead of meat or poultry with higher fat content can help keep blood cholesterol within normal levels.

Folic acid helps protect against birth defects, various forms of cancer and heart disease.

Vitamin B_1 aids in carbohydrate metabolism and is good for nerve function and growth.

Vitamin B_6 helps boost the immune system.

Potassium is essential for maintaining normal heart function and blood pressure.

Zinc aids in healing and is important for good reproductive health, especially for men.

PERSONAL ADVICE   A recent study reports that people suffering from psoriasis can find relief by eating a diet high in turkey. Researchers are not sure whether the turkey itself helps, or whether psoriasis victims may benefit from eating a low-fat diet.

Try hamburger and turkey hot dogs, which taste delicious and cut your fat consumption. Ground turkey is readily available in most markets and natural food stores.

Turnip (Greens)

FACTS If you've been eating the turnips but tossing away the greens, you're making a terrible mistake. Turnip greens are a terrific source of beta-carotene: one cup of cooked greens contains more than 150 percent of the RDA for this plant form of vitamin A. And speaking of antioxidants, turnip greens also contain about two thirds of the RDA for vitamin C.

The turnip bulb has no beta-carotene and half the amount of vitamin C. What it lacks in vitamins, however, it makes up in fiber. A half cup serving of cooked turnip bulb has nearly 5 grams of dietary fiber.

POSSIBLE BENEFITS Beta-carotene may help prevent many different forms of cancer and coronary artery disease.

Vitamin C is also believed to protect against cancer, and helps the body ward off infection.

The fiber in the turnip bulb helps maintain bowel regularity, which may help to prevent colon/rectal cancer.

Venison

FACTS At one time, in the not too distant past, venison (deer meat) was strictly for hunters. Today, it's featured on the menus of some of the best restaurants in the country. Why the change?

Venison is one of the healthiest meats around. It weighs in at a mere 1 gram of fat per ounce of meat—even the leanest cut of beef has twice the fat content. It is also low in calories (145 calories per 4-ounce serving) and is a reasonably good source of B vitamins, protein, and iron.

POSSIBLE BENEFITS By cutting the amount of saturated fat in your diet, you automatically reduce your risk of heart disease, strokes, and certain types of cancer.

B vitamins in general help convert food into energy and are essential for the normal functioning of the nervous system.

Iron can help prevent anemia.

PERSONAL ADVICE Venison can be ground up for hamburgers, grilled like steak, or made into stew. Be sure to buy venison from a good butcher, as some cuts can be very tough.

Watermelon

FACTS Picnics are synonymous with watermelon, and watermelon is synonymous with good health. One generous slice (about ¹⁄₁₆ of a large melon) contains a hefty dose of antioxidants vitamin C (about 80 percent of the RDA) and beta-carotene (about 30 percent of the RDA). It is also high in potassium and a good source of fiber.

POSSIBLE BENEFITS Vitamin C and beta-carotene may protect against various forms of cancer.

In their capacity as antioxidants, vitamin C and beta-carotene may help to prevent the oxidation of LDL cholesterol, which is believed to be responsible for the development of atherosclerosis. Potassium helps to regulate heart function and normalize blood pressure, which helps to prevent heart attack and stroke.

Fiber helps to maintain bowel regularity and prevent colon/rectal cancer.

Wheat Bran

FACTS There are lots of good reasons to include wheat bran as a daily part of your diet. It is high in insoluble fiber, the type that helps maintain bowel regularity. Eating a high-fiber meal will help you to feel fuller for a longer period of time than a low-fiber meal—that's because it takes the body longer to break down fiber than many other forms of carbohydrate. In addition, there is now some compelling evidence that wheat fiber may be a potent weapon against certain forms of cancer.

A case in point is colon cancer. Recently, scientists at New York Hospital/Cornell Medical Center studied 58 people with precancerous polyps, a condition that put them at greater risk of developing colon and rectal cancers. Half the group were put on a diet rich in wheat bran cereal. The others were given a low-fiber cereal. Four years later, researchers had good news for the group on the high-fiber wheat bran cereal—in many cases, their polyps had shrunk in size and number. Unfortunately, the polyps remained the same or grew for the people on the low-fiber diet.

Wheat bran may also prove to be a useful tool in preventing breast cancer. Many studies have found that women with breast cancer often have higher blood levels of certain forms of potent estrogens. Other studies have found that about one third of all breast tumors are estrogen-sensitive and, in fact, will shrink in size after antiestrogen therapy. Therefore, researchers believe that anything that helps reduce the blood levels of certain forms of potent estrogens may, in turn, help reduce the risk of breast cancer. A recent study sponsored by the American Health Foundation examined whether a high-fiber diet would help reduce blood estrogen levels. Sixty-two premenopausal women were divided into three groups: one group was given a diet high in oat bran, another group was given corn bran, and the third group was put on a diet rich in wheat bran. After two months, the women on the wheat bran diet showed a significant decline in serum estrone and estradiol, two forms of estrogen. The serum estrogens of the women on the corn and oat bran diets were unaffected.

On top of everything else, wheat bran is also a good source of B vitamins and provides some protein.

POSSIBLE BENEFITS May help prevent cancers of the colon and rectum.

May help reduce blood estrogen levels, thus preventing breast cancer.

B vitamins are necessary for the normal metabolism of food, among other important jobs.

CAUTION Vitamin B_6, which is found in wheat bran, may interfere with L-dopa, a drug used to treat Parkinson's disease. If you are taking L-dopa, do not use a bran product without first consulting with your physician.

PERSONAL ADVICE The wheat kernel includes three components: endosperm, germ, and bran. Processed wheat products, such as white flour, are made from only part of the wheat kernel and are much lower in fiber and nutrients than whole wheat flour. Good sources of wheat bran include products that are made out of whole wheat flour, and bran cereals.

Wheat Germ

FACTS Wheat germ, like the embryo of the wheat kernel, has a crunchy texture and a nutlike flavor. A mere 3 tablespoons of wheat germ provide 3.9 grams of dietary fiber, more than twice as much as in a slice of whole wheat bread. Wheat germ is also an excellent source of vitamin E, B vitamins (folic acid, niacin, thiamine), and selenium. In addition, wheat germ has a fair amount of zinc, phosphorus, and magnesium, each of which has an important role to play in maintaining normal body function.

A recent study published in the *Journal of Nutrition* (February, 1992) reports that people with high blood lipid levels may be able to significantly reduce cholesterol and triglycerides by eating between 20 and 30 grams (roughly 1 ounce) of raw wheat germ daily. Even better, wheat germ appears to cut LDL cholesterol but not the good HDL. Researchers suspect that wheat germ oil may prevent the oxidation of LDL cholesterol, which leads to the formation of plaque deposits in arteries, a leading cause of heart attack.

POSSIBLE BENEFITS As a rich source of fiber, wheat germ helps maintain bowel regularity and protect against rectal and colon cancer.

Raw wheat germ may protect against heart attack and stroke by reducing LDL cholesterol and triglycerides.

Vitamin E is an antioxidant that helps prevent various forms of cancer and heart disease.

Folic acid taken during pregnancy can help prevent neural tube defects. It also protects against cervical and other forms of cancer.

Selenium is an antioxidant that may help prevent many different forms of cancer.

Whole Wheat Pasta

FACTS At one time, it was practically a sacrilege to utter the words "pasta" and "diet" in the same breath. Today, more knowledgeable waist watchers know that pasta is one of the best ways to stay trim and fit. Pasta (except for egg noodles) is fat-free, high in complex carbohydrates, and low in calories. It is rich in nutrients such as B vitamins, potassium, and iron. Whole wheat pasta, which includes the wheat germ and bran, is also an excellent source of fiber—a ½-cup serving contains about 6 grams of dietary fiber.

POSSIBLE BENEFITS Fiber helps to maintain bowel regularity and may help to prevent colon and rectal cancer.

A low-fat diet helps prevent obesity, and may protect against various forms of cancer and heart disease.

Foods that are high in complex carbohydrates may help reduce the risk of diabetes in susceptible people by preventing sudden surges of glucose (blood sugar).

PERSONAL ADVICE Don't negate the health benefits of pasta by killing it with a high-fat, high-calorie sauce. Avoid sauces based in butter and cream; use a meatless tomato sauce or a light olive oil sauce with sautéed garlic or vegetables.

Wine

FACTS Since ancient times, wine has been valued for its medicinal properties. The Jewish Talmud says, "Wine is the foremost of all medicines." Wine was one of the earliest anesthetics and was also used as a disinfectant. In recent times, several studies have established a link between wine consumption and lower rates of coronary artery disease.

+ A leading French study showed that people who drank a half liter of red wine daily had higher levels of HDL or "good" cholesterol than those who did not.
+ Japanese researchers recently discovered an antifungal compound in grape skin called resveratrol that lowers the fat content in livers of rats, thus lowering overall cholesterol. Scientists suspect that resveratrol works the same way in humans.
+ A major study in the United States published in the prestigious scientific journal *Circulation* showed that women who drink one drink a day have higher levels of HDL or "good" cholesterol then those who abstain. (HDLs for the men in the study remained unchanged at one drink.)

Other studies confirm that moderate drinkers of alcohol in general, and wine in particular, have lower blood pressure and a lower incidence of coronary artery disease than those who don't drink.

Although researchers initially believed that only red wine offered any cardiovascular benefits, recent studies suggest that white wine may be just as effective.

POSSIBLE BENEFITS Moderate wine drinking appears to raise HDLs ("good" cholesterol) and provide protection against heart attack for both men and women.

CAUTION A little bit of wine may be good for the heart, but too much wine is poison, for your heart and other vital organs. People who average more than 1–2 drinks daily are at greater risk of developing cardiovascular problems such as high blood pressure and stroke. Scientists speculate that an excess of alcohol may interfere with the absorption of calcium, which is essential for normal blood pressure and heart function. Women take note: because alcohol may interfere with calcium absorption, women who drink more than 2 drinks a day run a greater risk of osteoporosis. Finally, there are some people who should not drink at all, notably those who are taking certain medications that may enhance the effect of alcohol, such as Valium, and people who are addicted to alcohol. Needless to say, drinking and driving don't mix.

PERSONAL ADVICE Red grape juice may offer many of the same benefits of red wine without the alcohol as a disadvantage. However, further studies need to be done before we can be sure.

Winter Squash

FACTS Move over carrots—winter squash, which is also rich in beta-carotene (more than 150 percent of the RDA), may be the better choice for maintaining good eyesight. A 12-year study of nurses at Harvard University showed that the women who ate fruits and vegetables rich in beta-carotene had a 39 percent lower risk of developing cataracts than those who did not. Winter squash (along with spinach and sweet potatoes) was among the strongest protectors— that is, women who remained cataract-free ate significantly more of these vegetables than women who developed cataracts. Oddly enough, women who ate the most carrots did not have a reduced risk of developing cataracts. Although the researchers were puzzled by this result, there is one possible explanation. Unlike carrots, winter squash (as well as spinach and sweet potato) is very high in potassium. Potassium, in turn, helps to prevent high blood pressure, which is also a major risk factor for developing cataracts. In sum, maybe it's the potassium that is the stronger protector, or the combination of beta-carotene and potassium.

Another good reason to eat winter squash—it has more than a third of the RDA for vitamin C. Vitamin C, an antioxidant, may also protect the eyes from the type of oxidative damage that may cause eye problems such as cataracts.

POSSIBLE BENEFITS Helps preserve normal eyesight.

Numerous studies confirm that people who eat foods rich in beta-carotene are at much lower risk of developing various forms of cancer.

A diet rich in beta-carotene appears to reduce the risk of developing coronary artery disease.

Vitamin C protects against cancer and heart disease and seems to help the body ward off viral infection.

Potassium helps maintain the normal fluid balance in the body, as well as normal blood pressure and heart function.

Yogurt

FACTS Here's more proof that the "old wives" really did know what they were talking about. For years, yogurt had been a popular folk remedy for vaginal yeast infections. Recently, a woman physician at Long Island Jewish Medical Center decided to investigate whether or not yogurt really worked. Dr. Eileen Hilton fed yogurt containing *Lactobacillus acidophilus* cultures for six months to women with a history of chronic yeast infections. (One in ten women suffer from chronic infections, which can occur as often as five or six times a year.) Her findings: Women who ate 8 ounces of yogurt each day had significantly fewer infections than those who did not.

Yogurt may also help the body ward off other types of infection. Dr. George M. Halpern, at the University of California at Davis, studied the effects of yogurt on the immune system. According to his research, people who ate daily two 8-ounce cartons of yogurt containing live cultures had higher blood levels of gamma-interferon, a substance that helps the body fight disease. He also discovered that the yogurt eaters had 25 percent fewer colds than nonyogurt eaters, and significantly fewer symptoms of hay fever and allergy.

Yogurt also provides a hefty amount of calcium. Plain, low-fat yogurt has about 45 percent of the RDA for this mineral. Fruited, nonfat yogurt has about 35 percent. It is also a good source of potassium, riboflavin, and B_{12}.

POSSIBLE BENEFITS Helps prevent vaginal yeast infection.
Helps bolster the immune system.
The calcium in yogurt helps maintain bone strength and prevent osteoporosis and can lower serum cholesterol.

Potassium helps to maintain normal blood pressure and heart function.

Riboflavin is essential for the conversion of food to energy.

B_{12} works with folic acid to help prevent anemia. B_{12} deficiency in older people can result in neurological symptoms that mimic Alzheimer's disease.

PERSONAL ADVICE The French eat 5 to 6 servings of yogurt daily, which might be the reason for their lower incidence of heart disease. Read the labels on the yogurt package very carefully.

Not all brands of yogurt have *L. acidophilus,* the only ingredient that has been shown to be useful against vaginal yeast infections. Be sure that you choose a low-fat or no-fat yogurt—the higher-fat yogurt offers more calories and less calcium.

A word about frozen yogurt: It may taste great, but it just doesn't have the same amount of active cultures. Low-fat or no-fat frozen yogurt, however, is still a better dessert choice than ice cream.

Foods to Watch

They may not be household names yet, but here are some foods that I predict you're going to be hearing a lot about in coming years.

Camu Camu

It's bigger than a cherry, has a sour flavor, and may be the hottest fruit yet to be imported from the Peruvian Amazon.

Why is this funny-sounding fruit so special? Camu camu is an amazing source of vitamin C; in fact, it contains up to thirty times the vitamin C found in citrus fruit. Vitamin C is a potent antioxidant and immune booster. Although it needs a little sweetening, this fruit can be made into juice, sorbet, or ice cream. Watch for it in your frozen-food case!

Flax

When we think of flax, we think of it as the source for linen and linseed oil; however, within the next few years, many of us will be eating this stuff and loving it. The National Cancer Institute is looking closely at flax for possible chemopreventive effects. Flaxseed is one of nature's richest sources of lignans (found in grains such as bran, buckwheat, and corn) and omega-3 polyunsaturated fatty acids (also found in fatty fish), two substances that can do a lot of good in the body. Lignans deactivate potent estrogens that can initiate the growth of cancerous tumors, especially in the breast and reproductive system. In fact, studies have shown that women who consume a diet high in lignans have lower rates of colon and breast cancer. Flax may offer double protection against cancer: omega-3 fatty acids appear to block the action of cancer-promoting prostaglandins. In addition, omega-3 fatty acids may help to prevent heart disease by lowering cholesterol and triglycerides in people with elevated blood lipids. A natural blood thinner, omega-3s may prevent dangerous blood clots, which can increase the risk of heart attack and stroke. Studies also show that omega-3 fatty acids may protect against inflammatory diseases, such as psoriasis, arthritis, and lupus, by altering the chemical pathway that can promote a flare-up of these conditions.

Until recently, flaxseed was ignored by food producers because it was quick to turn rancid, and can also interfere with the body's ability to use vitamin B_6. However, Paul Stitt, M.S., a biochemist in Wisconsin, developed a method of stabilizing flax and is now selling flax-enriched bread made by his company, Natural Oven bakeries in Manitowoc, Wisconsin. Stitt, who offers several delicious varieties of flax bread to Midwestern stores and through mail orders, is not interested in expanding his business, but is willing to teach all who want to come to Wisconsin how to bake this special bread so they can start their own local bakeries. (For more information, see Resources.)

Licorice

For thousands of years, Chinese healers have used licorice root to treat everything from ulcers to sore throats; in the Orient, it is highly regarded as a potent tonic for the heart and spleen. One of the early drugs in the treatment of ulcers, carbenoxolone, is actually a derivative of a compound in licorice. Here in the United States we are just beginning to take a closer look at the potential medicinal properties of this food.

Licorice root comes from a legume (like kidney beans and soybeans) and has a sweet flavor. Most of the candy sold in the United States as licorice is actually flavored with anise; however, in Europe, you can actually buy candy with a high licorice content. I believe that one day in the near future, some enterprising food manufacturer will bring out a line of licorice-enriched designer foods.

There are many reasons why the National Cancer Institute and other researchers are so interested in licorice these days. First, licorice root contains triterpenoids and phenolics, two compounds that may block cancer promotion. In addition, licorice contains glycyrrhizin, a compound that has been shown to have antibiotic activity against the bacteria that cause cavities. In fact, components of licorice root are already used in many mouthwashes.

CAUTION True licorice has a steroidlike effect on the body that can cause the retention of sodium and the depletion of potassium, which can result in high blood pressure. Therefore, people with high blood pressure should avoid eating licorice in any form. However, most people will not be harmed by a small amount of licorice.

Nuña

Soon we may all be saying, "What's a movie without a bag of nuñas?"

Nuñas, or pop beans, high in both fiber and protein, can be made into a tasty popcorn when heated in oil and popped in the microwave. These beans are grown in the Andes, but some enterprising Americans are looking for ways to grow them in the Pacific Northwest. Undoubtedly, nuñas will do well in a country that is starved for healthy snack food.

Purslane

Wait! Don't throw out that weed. It just may be the "super food" of the future.

Purslane, now considered a troublesome weed in the United States, is finding its way into the salads served in the best restaurants in Europe. According to the USDA, purslane, which has a mild, nutty taste and a crunchy texture similar to sprouts, contains more omega-3 fatty acids than any other plant studied to date, and is chock full of vitamin E. Both omega-3 fatty acids and vitamin E may provide protection against cancer, heart disease, and inflammatory diseases. This plant can grow practically anywhere, and I predict that it will soon pop up in your local greengrocery.

Food for Whatever Ails You

...

CHAPTER 5

Cooking Right

A garden-fresh carrot offers more than a day's supply of precious beta-carotene. A carrot that's been sitting on the grocer's shelf for several weeks contains only a fraction of that amount. The moral of this tale is, if you want to get the maximum benefit from your food, you're going to have to become an educated consumer.

First, you need to know what to shop for, and how to pick the good from the bad. Second, you need to know how to handle the food when you bring it home—even the best food can lose its potency if it's not stored properly. Finally, you need to know the correct way to prepare and cook food so that you preserve its vital nutrients.

Guidelines for Fruits and Vegetables

Buying Smart

The fresher the better: From the minute they're picked, fruits and vegetables begin to lose some of their vitamins—beta-carotene is particularly vulnerable to exposure to air and light. Try to get to the greengrocer or supermarket within one or two days of the arrival of produce.

Neatness counts: Buy only sun-ripened, fresh-looking, undamaged produce. Bruising or rough handling can destroy vitamins.

Avoid precut fruits or vegetables: Many supermarkets offer precut, prewashed vegetables and precut fruits such as melons or sliced pineapples, and it may seem convenient. However, convenience exacts a steep toll. These "fast" produce products are often sapped of too many vitamins and minerals that are lost in the preparations. Fruits and vegetables should be handled as little as possible before eating.

Storage Tips

A cool dry place: Store your produce in the refrigerator crisper or in airtight plastic bags. Don't cut up your fruits or vegetables into little pieces to make storage easier: doing so will increase their exposure to air which can destroy vitamins.

Avoid heat or sunlight: Certain foods, such as tomatoes, peaches, or pears, may need a day or two out of the refrigerator to ripen. Some foods, such as bananas and potatoes, should not be stored in the refrigerator at all. Place these fruits and vegetables in a cool area away from direct sunlight, which can destroy vitamins.

Prepare with Care

Rinse don't soak: Rinse your fruit and vegetables lightly under cool water just before eating. To avoid vitamin loss, don't immerse them in water.

Scrub don't peel . . . most of the time: As a rule, you should scrub your fruits and vegetables with a soft brush right before eating. In most cases, you don't want to peel produce because the peel is a good source of fiber and nutrients. However, unless you buy organically grown produce, there are times that you may want to peel. For example, apples and cucumbers are routinely sprayed and coated with a heavy wax, and you may not want to eat the skin. In addition, some scientists have recently warned that one of the chemicals used to prevent sprouts from forming on potatoes has not been properly tested on humans. In this case, peeling or eating around the skin may be your best bet. Don't worry about losing important vitamins or minerals, most of the nutrients in the potato are not even near the skin.

Cooking Tips

Easy does it: In general, eat your vegetables raw or al dente, that is, lightly cooked and crisp. Do not boil or overcook them.

Go light on the water: Since water-soluble vitamins (C, B-complex) and important minerals (potassium and selenium) can be lost in cooking fluid, use cooking methods that require the smallest amount of water possible, such as:

♦ Steaming is one of the best ways to conserve vitamins and minerals. To cook, cut vegetables into small, bite-size pieces and place in a steamer basket. (You can buy one at most hardware or housewares stores.) Put about ½ inch of water in a pot, place the basket inside the pot, cover, and let cook over a low flame. Most vegetables will take between 3 and 5 minutes; however, some such as Brussels sprouts will cook in about 10 minutes, and artichoke could take close to an hour.

♦ The microwave oven is also an excellent choice for cooking vegetables because it requires very little water and cooks food quickly. Cooking time may vary according to size and model of your oven. Check your manufacturer's microwave cookbook to see what works best in your particular oven. Only use microwave-safe containers; do not use empty margarine tubs or other plastic containers that were not designed to withstand high heat because they could melt and leach potentially carcinogenic chemicals into the food.

Go light on the fat: Never deep-fry vegetables—you lose important vitamins like beta-carotene, vitamins E and K. If you sauté vegetables, use only a tiny amount of oil, or better yet, moisten the pan with unsalted broth as needed. Stir-frying in a pan or wok is terrific because you only need to use a tablespoon or so of oil and the vegetables cook quickly.

No baking soda: Some people add a pinch of baking soda to brighten the color of vegetables. This process destroys B vitamins and C.

Frozen or Canned Fruits and Vegetables

If fresh produce isn't available, frozen or canned is an acceptable second choice. Here's some information that might come in handy.

Frozen-food tips: When buying frozen vegetables, make sure that the vegetables are not all clumped together in a solid block. You should actually be able to feel the individual peas, or the shape of the broccoli stalks through the package. If the package feels like an ice brick, put it back. In all likelihood, it's been thawed and refrozen, a process that can deal a lethal blow to important vitamins and minerals. Don't buy frozen vegetables drenched in butter or cream sauce—who needs the calories or the fat! Keep your freezer at 0 degrees Fahrenheit; higher temperatures can damage nutrients.

The microwave oven is great for frozen vegetables because they can be cooked in little or even no water. Check the directions on the package.

Canned vegetables: Buy canned vegetables with little or no added salt, sugar, or monosodium glutamate (MSG). Since some vitamins can be destroyed by high temperatures (vitamin C in particular), store cans in a cool, dry place. Heat canned vegetables slowly in their own liquid. Don't throw away the leftover fluid, it's filled with vitamins: Drink it or save it for cooking.

Tips for Cooking Meat, Fish, and Fowl

Meat: The fat content varies drastically among different cuts of meat. A moderate portion of rib roast can weigh in at 26 fat grams; a lean serving of bottom round is only 8 fat grams. Good meat choices include pork tenderloin, shoulder steak, and London broil.

Cooking meat, especially fatty meat, at very high temperatures can be dangerous to your health. Heat produces carcinogenic compounds called heterocyclic aromatic amines (HAAs). Barbecuing, a cooking method where food is exposed directly to flame, can spell double trouble. This cooking method produces polycyclic aromatic hydrocarbons (PAH) which occur in the smoke when the fat from the meat drips down into the coals. The carcinogenic fumes then drift up and coat the meat. Obviously, using leaner cuts of meat may help to eliminate this risk. In addition, partially cooking the meat in your oven or microwave before placing it on the grill may help eliminate some of the fat, and also can reduce the amount of time the meat is being cooked at intensely high temperatures over the hot coals.

Broiling under a very high flame in the oven can also produce PAH. To avoid cooking at excessively high temperatures, place your meat (or chicken or fish) in an unheated broiler. Cook your meat thoroughly, but don't cook the life out of it. Overcooking not only dries it out (and if you're eating a low-fat cut to begin with, it may make it too dry) but produces more of the carcinogenic substances.

Poultry: Chicken and turkey are relatively low in fat and excellent sources of iron, B vitamins, and other important nutrients. Poultry skin, however, is packed with fat; avoid it if you can. It is okay, however, to cook chicken or turkey with the skin on, and peel it off before you eat. Stick to white meat, which is lower in fat. Don't deep-fry chicken; you lose most of its health benefit. Bake, broil, or sauté in as little oil as possible. Baste with broth, lemon or orange juice.

Fish: Buy the freshest fish from a trustworthy supermarket or fish store. Make sure that the eyes are bright (if you select the whole fish) and there is no telltale "fishy" odor. Fresh fish has a mild odor at best. Bake, broil, poach, or lightly sauté fish in a small amount of oil (or use broth to prevent sticking to the pan). Season fish with wine, herbs, lemon juice, or low-sodium broth.

Food Safety Tips

Each year, 9000 Americans die from eating tainted food, and untold millions are made ill from food that has not been handled or processed properly. The following are some tips on how you and your family can avoid becoming casualties.

Thoroughly Cook Food

Cook all perishable foods at temperatures above 325 degrees—lower temperatures actually activate bacteria. Use a meat thermometer to make sure that beef and poultry are cooked through. The Center for Science in the Public Interest suggests cooking beef to 160 degrees, chicken to 185 degrees, and lamb, veal, and pork to 170. Given the prevalence of salmonella, do not eat raw eggs. Cook eggs until they are solid, not soft and runny. Avoid soft-boiled or sunny-side up.

Keep Perishables Cold

Milk, cheese, and meats are meccas for the microbes that cause food poisoning. Buy only pasteurized milk, and be sure that it is well refrigerated at the store. Refrigerate milk and milk products as soon as possible after shopping, don't let them sit in the car for hours on end. Keep a frozen-food chest in your car for meat and dairy if you're not going to be home within two hours. Turn your home refrigerator down to 40 degrees or less. Milk can spoil if you leave it out at room temperature for more than two hours. Quickly refrigerate cooked meats after serving them. Don't allow them to sit on the counter for more than an hour. If you're not sure whether something has become spoiled, throw it out to be on the safe side. Don't taste it, a tiny bite is all it takes to get food poisoning.

Raw Chicken: Handle with Great Care

Between one third and 90 percent of all chickens are tainted with salmonella, a dangerous bacterium that can cause severe food poisoning. Cooking the bird thoroughly will eliminaᵗe these bacteria, but you need to make sure that while you are handling the raw chicken, you don't need-lessly spread the bacteria throughout your kitchen. First, when you buy a chicken, wrap it in a protective plastic bag so that blood doesn't accidentally leak onto other food. Sec-ond, refrigerate chicken as soon as possible—don't let it sit in the car for more than an hour or so. Third, remember that everything that comes in contact with the chicken needs to be washed, preferably with an antibacterial soap. Be careful about reusing knives, cutting boards—or any-thing else that you may have used for the chicken—before thoroughly washing them. Don't forget to wash your hands after handling the chicken. If you marinate the chicken, boil the marinade before using it again on the cooked chicken, or to be extra safe, make a fresh one.

Free-range, organic chickens sold at specialty stores and butchers may be a more wholesome choice. Unlike other commercial poultry, they are not fed growth hormones or antibiotics. Although these birds are raised in an environ-ment that is less likely to breed infection, I would still exer-cise the greatest caution in handling any chicken, regardless of upbringing. I prefer to buy skinless chicken for two rea-sons: first, most of the fat is in the skin, and second, the skin is more likely to have come in contact with feces and dirt that can carry dangerous bacteria.

Something Fishy

Don't keep fresh fish for more than twenty hours in your refrigerator without cooking it. Thoroughly cook all fish—avoid eating raw clams, mussels, and oysters, which can carry dangerous parasites. If you eat sushi (which I don't advise), go only to restaurants that you know and trust.

Most of us can survive an attack of food poisoning; however, there are some groups that are particularly vulnerable. People with compromised immune systems—those with diseases such as AIDS, the elderly, and people who are chronically ill—may be more prone to certain forms of food poisoning. These people should not take any chances with their health: they should avoid any questionable food. In addition, children and fetuses are more likely to suffer serious side effects from food-borne diseases; therefore parents and mothers-to-be must be extra vigilant about sanitary conditions in their homes and in the other places where they or their children eat.

Eating Right:
From Three Squares to a Pyramid

Since the 1950s, the U.S. Department of Agriculture has advised Americans to eat three meals a day with hefty quantities from the four major food groups—dairy, meat, fruits and vegetables, and grains. To illustrate its point, the government used a pie cut into four equal pieces—with each piece representing a different food group—as a symbol of the well-balanced meal. As more and more research confirmed that the American diet was in large part responsible for the virtual epidemic of cancer and heart disease in this country, the USDA has finally replaced the pie with the Food Guide Pyramid designed to vividly show that not all foods are created equal.

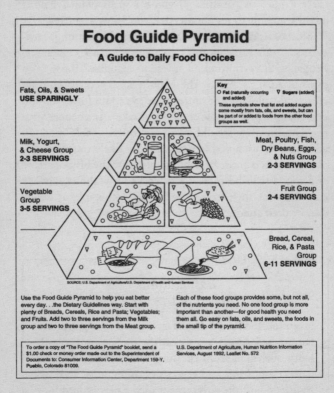

Food Guide Pyramid

A Guide to Daily Food Choices

Fats, Oils, & Sweets
USE SPARINGLY

Key
○ Fat (naturally occurring ▽ Sugars (added) and added)
These symbols show that fat and added sugars come mostly from fats, oils, and sweets, but can be part of or added to foods from the other food groups as well.

Milk, Yogurt, & Cheese Group
2-3 SERVINGS

Meat, Poultry, Fish, Dry Beans, Eggs, & Nuts Group
2-3 SERVINGS

Vegetable Group
3-5 SERVINGS

Fruit Group
2-4 SERVINGS

Bread, Cereal, Rice, & Pasta Group
6-11 SERVINGS

SOURCE: U.S. Department of Agriculture/U.S. Department of Health and Human Services

Use the Food Guide Pyramid to help you eat better every day. . .the Dietary Guidelines way. Start with plenty of Breads, Cereals, Rice and Pasta; Vegetables; and Fruits. Add two to three servings from the Milk group and two to three servings from the Meat group.

Each of these food groups provides some, but not all, of the nutrients you need. No one food group is more important than another—for good health you need them all. Go easy on fats, oils, and sweets, the foods in the small tip of the pyramid.

To order a copy of "The Food Guide Pyramid" booklet, send a $1.00 check or money order made out to the Superintendent of Documents to: Consumer Information Center, Department 159-Y, Pueblo, Colorado 81009.

U.S. Department of Agriculture, Human Nutrition Information Services, August 1992, Leaflet No. 572

Based on the new guidelines, here's what the average American is supposed to eat on a given day:

6–11 Servings of Bread, Cereal, Rice, and Pasta
   1 serving = 1 slice of bread or ½ cup of rice

2–4 Servings of Fruit
  1 serving = 1 medium fruit or 6 oz fresh
      fruit juice

3–5 Servings of Vegetables
  1 serving = 1 cup raw, leafy vegetables or 6
      oz vegetable juice

2–3 Servings of Dairy Foods
  1 serving = 1 cup yogurt or 1 cup milk or 1
      oz cheese

2–3 Servings of Meat, Fish, Poultry, Dry
      Beans, Eggs, and Nuts
  1 serving = 3 to 4 oz animal protein, roughly
      the size of a deck of cards, or ¼ cup nuts

Fats, at the very top of the pyramid, are to be used sparingly.

Experts agree that roughly 55 to 60 percent of food should be in the form of carbohydrates (grains, starches, fruits and vegetables). Fats should constitute no more than 30 percent of daily calories (the average intake in the United States is around 37 percent). Protein consumption should be limited, which will happen naturally if you watch your portion size of protein-rich foods, such as meat. Most Americans eat more than 100 grams of protein daily—twice as much as they actually need.

Salt intake should be limited to 2400 mg daily. This can be achieved by avoiding highly salted food and not adding additional salt to food.

CHAPTER 6

What to Feed a Cold and Other Ailments

Food can be powerful preventive medicine. The following section lists common ailments, and the foods, vitamins, or diet that may help to prevent them or relieve symptoms.

Acne

FACTS Acne, the bane of adolescence (which can also strike young adults), is caused by the overproduction of a substance called sebum, which is produced by the oil glands of hair follicles. When the pores become clogged with sebum, the result are the blackheads, pimples, and pustules that erupt on the face and chest.

Dietary Recommendations

Avoid iodine (salty foods). Eat foods rich in beta-carotene (sweet potato, green leafy vegetables, and apricots), zinc (oysters, wheat germ, beans), and acidophilus (yogurt).

At one time, it was thought that fatty foods can cause acne; however, that is no longer a widely held belief. In fact, salt may be the real culprit. Iodine, which is added to most table salt to prevent goiter, has been shown to trigger skin eruptions. Iodine is particularly abundant in processed food such as chips, fries, and fast-food burgers, which are often heavily salted. Teenagers who are worried about acne should stick to unrefined, unprocessed food and should avoid adding too much salt to their food. In addition, if an acne-prone teen takes a vitamin supplement, he or she should make sure that it is low in iodine.

Vitamin A is essential for healthy skin. In fact, Accutane, a potent form of synthetic vitamin A, is a common treatment for acne. (Accutane must be taken under a physician's supervision, and should never be used by pregnant women.) Vitamin A itself should never be taken in high doses; however, it's perfectly safe to load up on beta-carotene-rich foods, which can be converted to vitamin A as the body needs it. Teenagers should munch on carrots, dried apricots, sweet potatoes, spinach, broccoli, and other good sources of beta-carotene; these foods not only are good for their skin but will offer them a lifetime of protection against cancer and heart disease.

Zinc, which promotes healing, is also excellent for the skin. Eat oysters, beans, wheat germ, and other zinc-rich foods.

Acidophilus, the friendly bacterium found in yogurt, also helps to keep skin clear.

If the acne is severe, see a physician. There are many treatment options available today that can help clear up this condition.

Allergies

FACTS An allergy is caused by a hypersensitivity to an allergen—a food, cosmetic, or substance that is inhaled or worn—that triggers the production of histamine and serotonin, which, in turn, cause an inflammatory response. It's often very difficult to isolate exactly what you are allergic to; the culprit may be hidden in food in the form of additives, food coloring, and preservatives. However, if you do notice that you experience respiratory distress or develop a rash after eating a particular food, your best bet is to simply avoid it.

Dietary Recommendations

Eat onion, take vitamin C, B-complex, and bromelin supplements.

Researcher Eric Block, Ph.D., of the State University of New York, discovered a sulfur compound in onion that in test-tube studies can prevent the biochemical chain of events that lead to asthma and allergic reactions. Does this mean that eating onions will help prevent allergies in humans? Although there's no scientific proof, we do know that for thousands of years, Chinese healers have prescribed onion for respiratory problems, so there just may be something to the "onion treatment."

Vitamin C in doses over 2000 mg per day can trigger the release of antihistamines, which can help alleviate allergic symptoms. However, in some people, this dose of vitamin C can cause stomach cramps, dry nose, and diarrhea. Take 1000 mg of vitamin C twice daily after meals to minimize the risk of unpleasant side effects, but discontinue use if you develop any.

Bromelin, a compound extracted from pineapple, is also useful in alleviating allergic symptoms. Take 1 to 3 tablets daily.

Finally, a good B-complex supplement will help the body deal with the stress of allergy. Make sure the supplement contains at least 100 mg of pantothenic acid. Nutritional yeast is a fabulous source of B vitamins.

Anemia

FACTS Anemia is characterized by a deficiency in the number of red blood cells and/or a reduction in the number of hemoglobin molecules. Symptoms include fatigue, increased susceptibility to infection, and the inability to concentrate. In its more severe form, anemia can impair the supply of oxygen to body tissues, which can result in shortness of breath and extreme lethargy.

The most common cause of anemia is an inadequate supply of iron; however, that is not the only cause. A folic acid deficiency can also result in a reduced number of red blood cells. A lack of copper and vitamins B_6 and B_{12} can also interfere with the formation of red blood cells, but these causes of anemia are quite rare. Before a diagnosis of a specific type of anemia can be made, a physician needs to perform several blood tests.

Iron-deficiency anemia is more prevalent among premenopausal women, particularly those with a heavy menstrual flow.

Eating iron-rich foods will help prevent iron-deficiency

anemia. Don't wash your meals down with coffee or any other beverage with caffeine; it hampers iron absorption. Eat iron with vitamin C; it promotes absorption.

Dietary Recommendations

Eat foods rich in iron (red meat, dried fruit, fortified cereals, dried beans).

To prevent folic-acid-deficient anemia, eat yeast, wheat germ, dried beans, sunflower seeds, and an occasional piece of liver.

Arthritis

FACTS Arthritis, inflammation of one or more joints in the body, is characterized by stiffness, soreness, or pain in joints, especially upon waking in the morning, and by fatigue and weakness that cannot be attributed to another disorder. Some 20 million Americans suffer from arthritis—many more women than men.

Rheumatoid arthritis, a common form, is an autoimmune disease occurring when the body's own immune system attacks healthy tissue, destroying cartilage that connects joints.

Through the years, there have been many so-called diets and home remedies for arthritis. However, there are no cures, although there are several treatments that may be effective, depending on the severity of the condition. Many arthritics find relief with simple aspirin; others do well taking other nonsteroidal anti-inflammatory drugs.

Dietary Recommendations

Eat foods rich in omega-3 fatty acids (mackerel, albacore tuna, salmon).

Through the years, there have been many claims that diet can help arthritis. Some of the recommended diets have been strange and unsubstantiated by any serious research. As a result, many members of the medical community dismiss the entire notion that diet can affect arthritis. However, there is growing evidence that omega-3 fatty acids—the kind found in fish oil and flaxseed—can help alleviate arthritic symptoms. Several studies show that omega-3 fatty acids as a dietary supplement, along with anti-inflammatory drugs, can reduce arthritic stiffness and pain. Omega-3 fatty acids alter the chemical pathway that leads to the production of certain prostaglandins, hormonelike chemicals that trigger the inflammatory process. As a result, there is less inflammation and less pain.

PERSONAL ADVICE If you're taking aspirin on a regular basis to cope with arthritic symptoms, keep in mind that aspirin can sap your body of vitamin C. Make sure to eat lots of vitamin-C-rich foods. Eliminating nightshades (potato, eggplant, and tomato) from your diet may help diminish your arthritic symptoms.

Bladder Cancer

FACTS Bladder cancer, the most common malignant tumor of the urinary tract, is most prevalent among 50- to 70-year-olds. Close to 50,000 new cases are reported each year. Cigarette smoking and exposure to certain industrial chemicals greatly increase your risk of developing this form of cancer.

Dietary Recommendations

Eat foods rich in vitamin C (white potato, broccoli, asparagus), lycopene (ruby red grapefruit, tomato, red pepper), and beta-carotene (cantaloupe, kale, Romaine lettuce).

Several studies have shown that vitamin C inhibits the formation of nitrosamine in the mouth and digestive tract which can contribute to the growth of cancerous tumors in the bladder. Vitamin C also deactivates other carcinogens that could contribute to bladder cancer.

Other studies show that people with bladder cancer have lower blood levels of beta-carotene than people without this form of cancer. In addition, people with bladder cancer have lower than normal levels of lycopene, a carotenoid found in tomatoes, ruby red grapefruits, and red peppers.

Eating a wide range of fruits and vegetables should provide good beta-carotene and vitamin C protection against bladder cancer. In addition, people with chronic bladder infections may be at an increased risk of developing bladder cancer; therefore, be sure to see a physician if you have any symptoms, such as burning upon urination or blood in the urine, that could be a sign of infection. Generous amounts of cranberry juice will also help to prevent bacteria from sticking to the walls of the urinary tract, which could promote infection.

Bleeding Gums

FACTS Tender, bleeding gums can be a sign of gum disease, and anyone with this problem should see a dentist promptly. However, in many cases, bleeding gums are a result of a nutritional deficiency, specifically that of the bioflavonoid rutin, which helps to strengthen tiny blood vessels called capillaries. Rutin, along with other bioflavonoids, is added to C-complex supplements, and is present in many of the same foods that are rich in vitamin C.

Dietary Recommendations

Eat buckwheat (kasha) and citrus fruits (oranges, lemons, tangerines).

Bioflavonoids are present in plant food, specifically fruits, vegetables, nuts, and seeds. Rutin in particular is abundant in buckwheat or kasha. To treat your bleeding gums, eat more flavonoid-rich foods, and/or take a vitamin C-complex supplement with rutin.

Breast Cancer

FACTS Breast cancer is increasing at an alarming rate among women: in 1990, there were 150,000 new cases diagnosed. An estimated 44,000 women die from this disease each year. One out of nine women will get breast cancer. Vigilant self-examination and an annual mammogram past the age of 50 (or younger for women at high risk—that is, who have a mother, sister, or grandmother with breast cancer) are critical factors in preventing this kind of cancer. However, diet may also play a major role.

Dietary Recommendations

Eat foods rich in beta-carotene (mango, peach, spinach), omega-3 fatty acids (albacore tuna, sardines, bass), soy products (tofu, soybeans), vitamin C (citrus fruits, snow peas, Brussels sprouts), cruciferous vegetables (broccoli, cabbage, bok choy), and wheat bran.

Nature is filled with "medicines" that may help to prevent breast cancer.

Studies show that women with breast cancer tend to have low blood levels of beta-carotene and vitamin C. Eating more yellow and orange fruits and vegetables and green leafy vegetables, which are rich in both vitamin C and beta-carotene, may help to reduce your risk of breast cancer.

Women with breast cancer tend to have higher blood estrogen levels than normal. Estrogen can stimulate the growth of certain estrogen-sensitive tumors, particularly in the breast and reproductive system. Any substance that lowers or controls the amount of estrogen circulating in the bloodstream may be helpful in preventing certain forms of breast cancer. Indole, a compound found in cruciferous vegetables such as cabbage, broccoli, and Brussels sprouts, may prevent breast cancer by deactivating the estrogen compounds that promote tumor growth. Broccoli also contains sulforaphane, another compound that may block carcinogens from destroying healthy cells.

A recent study sponsored by the American Health Foundation found that women who eat wheat bran had lower levels of serum estrogens, which researchers believed reduced their risk of developing breast tumors.

Soybeans and soy products (soy milk, tofu, etc.) may also provide some protection against breast cancer. Oriental women, who tend to eat a lot of soy products, have 10 to 15 percent lower circulating estrogen levels than Caucasian women, and much lower rates of breast cancer. Soy contains isoflavones, two compounds that are converted in the body to an estrogenlike substance, ekuol. Ekuol deactivates a potent estrogen, estradiol, the mother compound for estrogen, inhibiting its ability to bind to estrogen-sensitive cells and promote tumor growth.

Limonene, a constituent of citrus oil, inhibited the growth of mammary tumors in laboratory rats. More studies are needed to see if it has the same effect on humans, but it's still a good idea to eat lots of oranges, grapefruits, and tangerines.

Several studies also show that omega-3 fatty acids, the kind that are found in fish oil and flaxseed oil, inhibit the growth of tumors in animals, including mammary tumors. In contrast, omega-3 fatty acids, the kind that are found in most polyunsaturated vegetable oils, form a substance called *trans*-fatty acids which appear to promote the growth of tumors.

Through the years, there has been a heated controversy over the effect of fat in the diet on the incidence of breast cancer. A major study involving thousands of nurses concluded that the level of fat in the diet made no difference in terms of the risk of developing breast cancer. However, a study in the *Journal of the National Cancer Institute* showed that fat intake may indeed make a difference in whether or not a woman with breast cancer has a recurrence. Researchers noted that women with estrogen-rich tumors who ate a diet high in fatty foods before surgery were more likely to suffer a second bout of breast cancer than those who had a less fatty diet. Saturated fat appeared to be a major culprit. Women with a history of breast cancer would be wise to limit their fat intake.

Cataracts

FACTS A cataract is an opaque covering that can form in the lens of the eye, typically in older people, and can result in blurred vision. Cataracts are one of the leading causes of blindness among the elderly.

Dietary Recommendations

Eat foods rich in beta-carotene (spinach, sweet potatoes, winter squash) and vitamin E (broccoli, almonds, wheat germ).

A 12-year study of nurses by researchers at Harvard University recently found that women who eat a lot of carotene-rich fruits and vegetables have a 39 percent lower risk of developing serious cataracts than those who don't. The foods that seem to offer the best protection against cataracts are spinach, sweet potato, and winter squash (all in the Hot Hundred). Researchers suspect that a carotene may protect against oxidative damage to the lens protein in the eye. Interestingly enough, carrots, which are high in beta-carotene, didn't even make it on the list of protective foods, which led researchers to speculate that perhaps a carotene different from beta-carotene is responsible for cataract prevention.

However, spinach, sweet potato, and winter squash are also rich in beta-carotene, so until more research is done, the answer to this question will remain a mystery.

Another study, this one by Finnish researchers, found that people with low levels of beta-carotene and vitamin E are nearly twice as likely to develop cataracts as people with high levels. Both vitamin E and beta-carotene are antioxidants, which prevent free radicals from causing damage to eye cells.

Cervical Cancer

FACTS The American Cancer Society estimates that there are roughly 13,500 new cases of cervical cancer each year in the United States, accounting for approximately 6000 deaths. Thanks to the Pap smear, most cases are caught early and the prognosis is good. However, prevention is still the best medicine, and diet may be a potent weapon against this form of cancer.

Dietary Recommendations

Eat foods rich in beta-carotene (sweet potato, carrots, kale), lycopene (ruby red grapefruit, red pepper, tomato), folic acid (asparagus, spinach, wheat germ), and vitamin C (cantaloupe, cauliflower, berries).

A major study of cervical cancer done in four Latin American countries shows that women with the lowest blood levels of beta-carotene are more likely to get cervical cancer than women with the highest levels. This study also showed that vitamin C may have a protective effect against cervical cancer. Eat lots of orange and yellow fruits and vegetables and green leafy vegetables, and you'll get a good amount of both vitamins.

A study from the School of Public Health at the University of Illinois at Chicago shows a link between blood levels of lycopene, a carotenoid found in foods such as tomato and ruby red grapefruit, and cervical cancer. Women with the lowest levels of lycopene were more likely to show early signs of cervical cancer than those with higher levels.

Folic acid also seems to play a protective role in cervical cancer. University of Alabama researchers compared 294 women diagnosed with cervical dysplasia, a precancerous condition. They found that those with the lowest levels of folic acid were most likely to develop abnormal cells. The researchers believe that folic acid may somehow protect against the HPV-16 virus, which sometimes leads to cervical cancer. Yeast, dried beans, spinach, asparagus, wheat germ, and sunflower seeds are good sources of folic acid.

Colon/Rectal Cancer

FACTS In Africa, cancer of the colon and rectum is a rare disease; in the United States, it is a virtual epidemic. According to the American Cancer Society, in 1990, there were 155,000 new cases of colon and rectal cancer diagnosed in the United States, and some 61,000 deaths due to this disease. Although genetics appears to play a role in some of these cases, only 8 percent of all cancers are linked to hereditary factors. In fact, many experts believe that diet may be the primary culprit.

Dietary Recommendations

Eat less fat, more fruits and vegetables, more foods rich
in folic acid (dried beans, wheat germ, asparagus) and
calcium (nonfat dairy products, sardines with bones, tofu
with calcium sulfate). Avoid pickled, cured, or smoked
foods.

Several epidemiological studies show that a high-fat diet
appears to increase the risk of developing this form of cancer. Researchers at the Harvard School of Public Health
examined the diets of more than 7000 men. Their findings:
those who consumed the highest amount of saturated fat
and the lowest in fiber were four times as likely to develop
colon polyps (often a prelude to cancer) as those who ate
diets high in fiber and low in fat. Why is fat harmful? Fat
stimulates the release of bile acids from the gallbladder. Fat
and bile travel through the intestinal tract into the colon,
where bacteria convert the bile acids into substances known
as secondary bile acids. Secondary bile acids are cocarcinogens, that is, they can produce changes in the cells in the
intestinal walls that can promote cancer.

Eating more insoluble fiber (from bran, fruits and vegetables, and legumes) will also help keep you cancer-free.
Fiber speeds up the amount of time food spends in the
digestive tract, thus reducing exposure to certain naturally
occurring carcinogens. Fiber also binds to bile acids, which
prevents them from irritating the colon wall.

Several studies show that people who eat a diet rich in
fruits and vegetables are at a much lower risk of developing
colon and rectal cancer. These foods not only are good

sources of fiber, but are also rich in beta-carotene and other protective phytochemicals.

Folate (folic acid) may also protect against this and other forms of cancer. Researchers took a dietary survey of 372 people with rectal cancer and 372 people who were cancer-free. The people who were cancer-free ate more folate-rich foods than people who developed rectal cancer. Food sources of folate include green leafy vegetables like spinach and asparagus.

Calcium also appears to play a protective role for colon and rectal cancer. A recent Finnish study shows that increasing calcium intake lowered the rate of cell turnover in the colon dramatically. Test-tube studies show that calcium binds (similar to fiber) to bile acids. Good sources of calcium include low- or no-fat dairy products, kale, and salmon with bones.

Salt-cured, pickled, or smoked foods can form carcinogenic compounds in the body that promote the growth of tumors in the digestive tract.

Common Cold

FACTS A cold is a viral infection that causes inflammation of the mucous membranes of the nose, throat, and bronchial tubes. The average cold lasts for about a week and, depending on its severity, can result in a sore throat, headache, achiness, runny nose, and cough.

One of the great ironies of modern medicine is that we can cure many complicated, life-threatening diseases, but we cannot cure the common cold, nor have we devised a shot to prevent it. Colds are caused by so many different viruses that once you develop an immunity against one, another one pops up. The average person gets between three to six colds a year, but there are things you can do to tip the odds in your favor.

Dietary Recommendations

Eat foods rich in vitamin C (strawberry, orange, cantaloupe), zinc (oysters, wheat germ, lamb chops), hot pepper, and chicken soup.

Your best line of defense against a viral infection is a strong immune system. Eating a well-rounded diet, with foods rich in natural immune boosters like vitamins A, C, E, and B_6 will increase your resistance against infection. Also keep in mind that anemia will reduce your ability to fight off a cold or any other infection, so be sure to get enough iron (meat, beans, and dried fruit) and folic acid (wheat germ, pumpkin seeds, asparagus) in your diet.

Once you get a cold, vitamin C will help lessen the cold's severity and duration. Eat lots of C-rich foods (mostly fruits and vegetables, including sweet red pepper, orange juice, broccoli, cantaloupe, grapefruit, cauliflower, mango, etc.). I normally take 1000 mg of vitamin C complex twice daily; however, when I feel a cold coming on, I increase the dose to 1000 mg every hour for a day or so. I recommend taking an esterified, time-release vitamin C complex—it's the gentlest on your stomach.

When you have a cold, think hot chili peppers. Hot peppers are a terrific decongestant. Load up on Szechuan or Mexican cuisine!

Hot chicken soup will also help to break up the mucus

that can cause congestion. (In many hospitals, chicken soup therapy is used as a legitimate treatment for pneumonia, along with other therapies.) In addition, chicken soup may have a mild antibiotic effect against infection.

Last, but not least, zinc lozenges, which are sold in many pharmacies and natural food stores, can in many cases help reduce the symptoms associated with a cold, and get you well faster. Zinc only works if you take it early in the cold. Suck (don't chew) one zinc lozenge (15 mg) every two hours, up to four times a day. Don't take zinc on an empty stomach.

Constipation

FACTS Constipation is characterized by hard stool that is difficult to pass, or when bowel evacuation is too infrequent for comfort. From commercials on television, you would be led to believe that laxatives are the only cure for this condition; in fact, diet is the best approach.

Dietary Recommendations

Eat insoluble fiber (celery, wheat bran, psyllium, pinto beans), and drink lots of water.

Foods rich in insoluble fiber will speed up food through the intestine. (Try to eat between 20 to 40 grams of fiber daily; at least half should be insoluble fiber.)

Drinking 8 glasses of water daily will help soften stool.

In general, eat more fruits and vegetables. Avoid heavily processed foods that have been stripped of their fiber.

Choose whole grain breads over white bread, eat brown rice instead of white rice, eat a bran muffin instead of a blueberry muffin made from white flour.

Getting more exercise will also help to keep your body regular.

Try to avoid over-the-counter laxatives; your body can become dependent on them, and they can also drain you of vital nutrients.

Coronary Artery Disease (Atherosclerosis)

FACTS Coronary artery disease (CAD) is a condition that occurs when the arteries carrying blood to the heart become narrowed or blocked entirely by deposits of plaque, a thick, yellowish, waxy substance. Plaque consists of cholesterol, a fat or lipid that is produced in the liver, as well as many different types of cells. When the flow of blood is cut off to the heart, the result is a heart attack.

Heart disease is the number-one killer in the United States, but there are many things that you can do to prevent it. First, you reduce your risk of having a heart attack by maintaining normal blood levels of cholesterol and triglycerides. Ideally, cholesterol levels should be below 200 mg/dl. More important, you should have a good ratio between LDL (low-density lipoprotein) or "bad" cholesterol (LDL carries cholesterol throughout the bloodstream) and HDL or "good" cholesterol; HDL (high-density lipoprotein) carries cholesterol to the liver for secretion in the bile. To ensure the right amount of each type of cholesterol, the ratio between total cholesterol and HDL should not exceed

6 : 1. Therefore, if your total cholesterol is 240, HDL should be 40 or more.

Triglycerides are another lipid well worth watching. For women, triglycerides over 190 mg/dl put them at a substantially higher risk of having a heart attack; for men, levels of 400-plus are a sign of potential danger.

Stress and a sedentary life-style are major risk factors for CAD. Diet, however, can be a powerful tool in preventing heart disease.

Dietary Recommendations

Eat a low-fat, high-fiber diet (fruits, vegetables, whole grains) with omega-3 fatty acids (mackerel, salmon, albacore tuna) and antioxidants (broccoli, carrots, citrus fruits).

The high-fat American diet is a major culprit in heart disease. Eating high amounts of cholesterol-rich food will increase blood cholesterol levels. So will eating high amounts of saturated fat, the kind found in meat and whole-fat dairy products, promote the production of cholesterol in the body. Therefore, the American Heart Association recommends reducing your intake of fat to no more than 30 percent of your total daily calories, with only 10 percent of that amount in the form of saturated fat. I suggest that you try to keep your fat intake to around 25 percent. In addition, keep your total cholesterol intake to under 300 mg per day.

Certain fats are better than others. Polyunsaturated fats, such as safflower oil, corn oil, or sunflower oil, may actually help to reduce cholesterol when used instead of saturated fat. However, at 9 calories per gram, any form of fat is fattening; therefore, do not add more than 2 to 3 teaspoons of polyunsaturated fat to your food daily.

Margarine, however, is another story. The process that turns oil into margarine can create *trans*-fatty acids, which can also promote the formation of cholesterol in the body. Tub margarine contains less *trans*-fatty acids than stick margarine; diet margarine contains even less. If you do use margarine, use it sparingly.

Many studies have shown that monounsaturated fats, especially the kind found in canola and olive oil, can lower cholesterol without lowering the beneficial HDL. Sprinkling 2 to 3 teaspoons of olive oil on your salad or vegetables daily is all you need to reap the maximum benefit.

Omega-3 fatty acids, found in fish such as mackerel, anchovy, white-meat tuna, halibut, salmon, and sardines, can also lower cholesterol and triglycerides in people with moderately elevated cholesterol and triglycerides. According to the National Heart and Lung Institute, a mere 1.0 gram of omega-3 fatty acids daily can significantly reduce heart disease, in men by 40 percent (and probably in women too, but until recently, they were excluded from many studies). To give you an idea of just how much fish you need to eat to get this amount, a 4-ounce serving of Atlantic salmon has more than 2 grams of fatty acid; a 4-ounce serving of tuna has 0.8 gram.

Certain vitamins are believed to reduce the risk of CAD. Antioxidants (beta-carotene, vitamins C and E, and selenium) prevent the oxidation of LDL or "bad" cholesterol, which may lead to the formation of plaque.

Carrots, which are rich in beta-carotene and calcium pectate, a type of fiber that lowers cholesterol, are a good choice for cholesterol watchers. In fact, according to a USDA study, eating two carrots a day can reduce cholesterol by as much as 20 percent. Foods rich in antioxidants include broccoli, bok choy, papaya, cantaloupe, citrus fruits, and green leafy vegetables.

Soluble fiber is a terrific cholesterol buster. It can be found in oat bran, apples, psyllium, barley, and legumes.

Many studies have shown that garlic, raw or cooked, can lower cholesterol, especially LDL cholesterol. Roast it, sauté it in olive oil, grate it into salad dressing—this stuff is good for your arteries.

Other foods that lower cholesterol include:

♦ Prunes lower LDL cholesterol.
♦ Alfalfa sprouts lower cholesterol in people with elevated cholesterol levels.
♦ Cucumbers contain a compound called sterol in their skin, which lowers cholesterol.
♦ Chili peppers contain capsaicin, a substance that reduces cholesterol and triglycerides.
♦ Green tea contains catechins, which lower cholesterol in animal studies.
♦ Grapes and wine contain resveratrol, which reduces cholesterol.

If diet alone doesn't work, consider taking a vitamin supplement. B vitamins niacin and pantothenine, a metabolite of pantothenic acid, are potent cholesterol busters that also cut triglycerides. Chromium has also been shown to cut triglycerides. Talk to your physician about which supplement would be best for you.

Diabetes Mellitus

FACTS Diabetes mellitus is an umbrella term used to describe several different but related metabolic disorders that afflict up to 14 million Americans and are the seventh leading cause of death in the United States. Women are nearly twice as likely to develop diabetes as men are. If untreated, diabetes can lead to serious complications including heart attack, stroke, kidney disease, and blindness. In general, diabetic disorders are characterized by hyperglycemia, high concentrations of glucose or blood sugar. The abnormally high glucose concentrations may be caused by an inadequate amount of insulin (the hormone that gets blood glucose into body cells where it fuels many important body functions) or by the body's inability to respond properly to the insulin it produces, which is known as insulin resistance. Type I or insulin-dependent diabetes (formerly called juvenile diabetes) is caused by the inability of the pancreas to produce any insulin at all. Type I diabetes usually strikes suddenly and dramatically before age 40. People with this form of diabetes must take insulin to maintain normal sugar levels. Type II diabetes, also known as adult or late-onset diabetes, accounts for 90 percent of all cases of diabetes and occurs during or after middle age. Very often, there are no symptoms; typically a physician first detects the problem when a patient displays an elevated fasting blood glucose level after a routine physical. There appears to be a genetic tendency to develop diabetes, although obesity is a major risk factor. In fact, between 80 and 90 percent of people with Type II diabetes are overweight.

People with diabetes are often put on high-carbohydrate, high-fiber diets; their sugar intake is severely restricted.

Dietary Recommendations

Eat foods rich in fiber and complex carbohydrates (fruits, vegetables, legumes, whole grains), spices (cinnamon, clove, bayleaf), and chromium (broccoli, grapefruit, shellfish).

Many physicians also believe that diet may play an important role in the prevention of Type II diabetes. As we age, our bodies become less able to use insulin efficiently; therefore, it's important to design your daily diet to prevent any sudden peaks or rises in blood sugar. Complex carbohydrates (especially grains and legumes) that burn slowly and steadily are good food choices that give insulin the time it needs to utilize glucose. Based on studies by fiber maven James W. Anderson, M.D., of the HCF Nutrition Foundation in Lexington, Kentucky, fiber also improves blood glucose and lipid levels in diabetics. (By the way, I'm not saying that an occasional chocolate bar, sugary dessert, or low-fiber meal is going to bring on diabetes, but a constant diet of sweets may contribute to the onset of insulin resistance, as well as obesity.) Certain foods also appear to enhance insulin's efficiency. According to studies performed by the USDA's Dr. Richard Anderson, spices such as cinnamon, clove, bay leaf, and turmeric may triple insulin's ability to metabolize glucose.

Chromium, a trace mineral, also appears to play an important role in helping the body use glucose. According to another USDA-sponsored study by Dr. Richard Anderson, rats fed a chromium-deficient diet produced nearly half the amount of insulin as rats fed a chromium-sufficient diet, when stimulated by a glucose solution. There is no RDA for chromium; however, experts recommend between 50 to 200 mcg for adults daily. According to the USDA, few Americans get enough of this mineral, which is found in brewer's yeast, broccoli, ham, grape juice, and shellfish.

CAUTION Anyone who is diabetic needs to be under a physician's care.

Diarrhea

FACTS Diarrhea—stool that is too watery or comes too often—is usually caused by nothing more serious than a mild bacterial or viral infection and goes away on its own within a day or two. Very often, medication to stop the diarrhea not only is unnecessary but can be counterproductive: diarrhea is your body's way of fighting against the invaders. There is a risk, however, of losing too much fluid and important minerals that may throw your body chemistry out of whack. Therefore, a careful diet is essential during this time of stress.

Dietary Recommendations

Drink clear fluids and juices, eat lightly, concentrate on pectin-rich foods (blueberries, apples, bananas) and replace the lost potassium (banana).

As your body loses fluid and potassium, you may begin to feel a bit tired and "washed out." Drink lots of clear broth, water, weak herbal tea, and ginger ale (which is especially good if you're also nauseous) to replace the lost liquid. Coke or Coke syrup may also help to reduce the amount of diarrhea.

Pectin, a form of soluble fiber found in some foods, including apple, carrot, and rice, can help relieve diarrhea by absorbing water and irritants in the bowel. (A grated raw apple with skin or grated carrot is a traditional remedy for this ailment.) Banana is also terrific because it not only is a source of pectin, but contains potassium, which is being leached from the body.

Blueberries contain special compounds which can help stop diarrhea (and also some potassium).

If the diarrhea continues for more than two days, or if there is any blood in your stool, immediately call your physician. It could be a sign of a more serious medical problem.

Diverticulosis

FACTS Diverticulosis is marked by the presence of diverticula, saclike herniations that can form in any part of the gastrointestinal tract, but usually crop up in the colon. This condition, which may go unnoticed for years, is often diagnosed after a barium enema. If the diverticula became inflamed, the result is diverticulitis, a condition that can cause cramps and lead to intestinal obstruction. Diverticulosis is common among older people with a history of constipation; common sense dictates that it can be avoided by eating a diet that promotes bowel regularity.

Anything that improves the motility of food through the digestive tract will help prevent diverticulosis (and most gastrointestinal cancers). Once diverticulosis is diagnosed, a

Dietary Recommendations

Eat bran (whole grain cereals), fiber (fruits, vegetables, whole grains, legumes), and drink fluids.

---

high-fiber diet will help prevent the kind of inflammation that leads to diverticulitis. Wheat bran and other forms of insoluble fiber will help maintain bowel regularity. Water will help soften the stool and keep things moving along. Diverticulitis, however, is treated quite differently; patients are put on antibiotics and fed a *low*-fiber diet. Anyone with this problem must be treated by a physician, since severe cases could lead to a rupture of the colon.

Gout

FACTS   Gout, a form of arthritis, is characterized by an excess of uric acid in the blood, which results in the formation of crystal-like deposits in the joints which can lead to pain and swelling, especially in the big toe. Some 2 million Americans suffer from gout; although gout is hereditary, excessive weight gain can speed up the onset of this disease. A combination of diet and medication can help to control it.

Dietary Recommendations

Avoid foods high in purines (organ meats), drink lots of water.

Gout is treated with a drug called allopurinol, which controls the rate at which the body produces uric acid. Eliminating certain foods from your diet—foods that are high in purines—can also help to relieve gout symptoms, since the body converts purines into uric acid. Foods that are rich in purines include organ meats such as kidney, liver, and sweetbreads (all very high in cholesterol), mackerel, and dried legumes. In addition, drinking 6 to 8 glasses of water a day can help flush the uric acid from your body, and may also help prevent another problem related to gout—the formation of kidney stones.

Hay Fever

FACTS   Hay fever is caused by a sensitivity to pollen, which triggers an allergic reaction. The body's immune system attempts to ward off the allergen by producing antibodies to attack it. Chemicals called histamines are released into the bloodstream. The result: a stuffy nose, watery eyes, and general discomfort.

Dietary Recommendations

Take vitamin C supplement.

In this case, a vitamin supplement may be useful. Studies have shown that high levels of vitamin C can lower histamine levels in the body up to 40 percent, which will reduce the discomfort of hay fever. To ward off a hay fever attack, try taking 1000 mg of vitamin C twice daily for two weeks. Some people may experience stomach upset or dry nose at these levels; if so, discontinue use. The calcium ascorbate form of vitamin C should eliminate this problem.

Headache

FACTS Just about everybody has had a headache at one time or another, although some people get them more often and in a more severe form. There are many different types of headaches which can be caused by many different things. PMS headaches are a result of monthly hormonal swings in women; nervous tension headaches are from stress; and migraine headaches, which are genetic, occur when the blood vessels in the brain become dilated. For some unknown reason, migraines afflict many more women than men. For some people, certain foods trigger headaches. Chocolate, caffeinated beverages, red wine, smoked meats, cheddar cheese, and monosodium glutamate (MSG), a common food additive, are known culprits. Obviously, if you notice that you come down with a headache after eating a particular food, avoidance is your best strategy.

Dietary Recommendations

Eat foods rich in magnesium (nuts, leafy vegetables) and calcium (nonfat dairy products, sardines with bones, almonds) and take an antistress B vitamin. Drink a cup of soothing peppermint tea.

Calcium and magnesium, both effective against PMS, another stress-related disorder, are also good for preventing headaches. A recent study reported in *Headache* magazine showed that women who take 200 mg of calcium daily have significantly fewer headaches than those who don't, especially during their periods. Yogurt, tofu with calcium sulfate, and almonds are good sources of calcium.

If you eat a lot of nuts, seeds, and green vegetables, or live in an area with hard water, you're probably getting enough magnesium. However, if you don't, it's easy not to get enough magnesium. You are at particular risk if you drink alcohol frequently or use diuretics ("water pills") or if you're a woman on supplemental estrogens. Other good food sources of magnesium are milk, bananas, wheat bran, apricots, and curry powder.

If your diet is low in magnesium-rich foods, and you are plagued by premenstrual headaches, try taking a calcium/magnesium supplement (500 mg magnesium to 250 mg calcium) seven to ten days before your period until the onset of menstruation.

If you feel that your headaches may be stress-related, try taking an antistress B vitamin. The B family is especially good for combatting anxiety and irritability.

Finally, if you feel a headache coming on, try a home remedy that works for me. Make yourself a strong cup of peppermint tea, sit down in a comfortable chair, sip the tea slowly and *relax*. Very often, this will hold the headache at bay.

CAUTION Calcium and magnesium work together in the body: you need to take in twice as much calcium as magnesium. Too much magnesium can cause diarrhea and impaired kidney function, so do not exceed 1000 mg daily. (Please note that for PMS, women need to take twice as much magnesium as calcium.)

Hemorrhoids

FACTS Hemorrhoids, also called piles, are actually varicose veins in the area of the anus and the rectum. Half of all adults over fifty have hemorrhoids; they are often caused by obesity or chronic constipation and may be brought on by pregnancy. When it comes to hemorrhoids, the refined and processed American diet is a major culprit.

Dietary Recommendations

Eat bran (whole grains, wheat germ) and fiber (fruits, vegetables, whole grains, legumes), drink lots of water, avoid hot chili peppers.

Diet can go a long way in controlling the burning and itching of hemorrhoids. Adding 1 tablespoon of unprocessed bran to your food three times a day can help keep you regular and so will increasing your intake of fruits, vegetables, and whole grains. Drinking lots of water will help soften the stool, which will help prevent the kind of straining that can lead to a hemorrhoidal flare-up. If you're bothered by hemorrhoids, pass on the hot chili peppers, as they can be quite irritating. Also, caffeine-containing beverages such as coffee, chocolate, cola, and cocoa can promote itching and burning.

Vitamin E oil (used externally) can help reduce irritation. Apply the oil to the infected area with a cotton swab.

CAUTION Some people may be allergic to vitamin E oil. Therefore, before using it, try putting a tiny amount on your arm, and watch for itching or irritation. If you have pain or rectal bleeding, see your physician.

High Blood Pressure (Hypertension)

FACTS Blood pressure measures the force exerted by blood against the arterial wall. The top number measures the systolic pressure, which is generated when the heart contracts and pushes blood into the arteries. The bottom number measures the diastolic pressure, or the pressure of the arteries when the heart muscle relaxes between beats. Normal blood pressure is 120/80. Pressures over that number are considered borderline high. One in six American adults have bona fide high blood pressure—that is, a systolic pressure over 140 and a diastolic pressure over 90. Even a slightly elevated blood pressure can increase your risk of having a heart attack or stroke and should not be ignored.

Being overweight increases the odds that you will develop high blood pressure. Therefore, maintaining your normal weight is essential. Food can also play a role in helping to keep your blood pressure within normal limits.

Dietary Recommendations

Eat foods rich in omega-3 fatty acids (albacore tuna, sardines, sea bass), vitamin C (papaya, cantaloupe, berries), calcium (nonfat dairy products, almonds, broccoli), magnesium (nuts, leafy green vegetables), potassium (banana, white potato, yogurt) and cruciferous vegetables (broccoli, kale, Brussels sprouts). Also, eat garlic and celery.

Omega-3 fatty acids—the kind that are found in fatty fish and flaxseed oil—lower the level of thromboxane, a substance that is produced by the body and causes blood vessels to constrict. Elevated thromboxane levels are linked to high blood pressure.

A recent study from the Harvard School of Public Health showed that people who ate a diet high in fruit fiber had lower systolic blood pressures than people who did not. (Other forms of fiber were not as significant.) In addition, the study showed that higher levels of magnesium intake were associated with lower levels of blood pressure. Magnesium is also found in fruits and vegetables.

Garlic and cruciferous vegetables (broccoli, cabbage, kale) contain sulfide compounds which also lower blood pressure.

Celery contains a compound called 3-butylphthalide which reduces blood pressure in laboratory rats. The Chinese have been using it for centuries to treat high blood pressure.

Vitamin C has also been used effectively to lower blood pressure. According to one study published in *Nutrition Review,* 20 women given 1000 mg of vitamin C daily experienced a significant drop in their systolic pressure; 12 of those women were borderline hypertensive.

Calcium also significantly lowers blood pressure in human and animal studies. According to the Framingham Children's Study, children who ate the most calicum-rich foods, such as dairy products, had the lowest systolic pressures.

Potassium plays a major role in the body in normalizing blood pressure. According to one major study, patients on high blood pressure medicine could significantly reduce the amount of medication needed by adding potassium-rich foods to their diet. Foods that are rich in potassium include low-fat plain yogurt (also an excellent source of calcium), white potato, dried apricots, cantaloupe, banana, and orange juice. One word of warning: people with kidney disorders should not take a potassium supplement or eat a diet high in potassium.

Sodium chloride, or table salt, will raise blood pressure in salt-sensitive individuals. The American Heart Association recommends that you restrict your salt intake to around 2000 mg per day.

Kidney Stones

FACTS The kidneys filter waste products from blood. Kidney stones (usually made of calcium) are obstructions that can cause inflammation and damage. Roughly 10 percent of all men and 3 percent of all women will develop kidney stones.

Until recently, people with kidney stones were told to steer clear of calcium-rich foods. However, a recent study at Harvard School of Public Health suggests that this advice may be all wrong. During the four-year study, researchers monitored the diets of 45,619 men without kidney stones. Roughly 500 of these men eventually developed kidney stones. Interestingly enough, those who ate the least amount of calcium were at much greater risk to develop kidney stones than those who ate a diet high in calcium. Researchers speculate that calcium may interfere with the absorption of oxalate, a substance in foods such as spinach and rhubarb which has also been associated with the formation of kidney stones.

The study also revealed that men with the highest intake of fruits and vegetables, which are high in potassium, had half the risk of developing kidney stones.

Dietary Recommendations

Eat foods rich in potassium (dried apricot, yogurt, orange juice), calcium (nonfat dairy products, almonds, sardines with bones), drink lots of water and eat less animal protein.

Eating five servings a day of fruits and vegetables may help prevent kidney stones. Good sources of potassium include dried apricots, white potato, banana, lima beans, orange juice, and low-fat yogurt, which is also an excellent source of calcium.

Drinking lots of fluid may reduce your risk of developing kidney stones by close to 30 percent.

Eating large quantities of meat or other forms of animal protein appears to increase the odds of developing this problem. Magnesium found in dark green leafy vegetables may also help to prevent kidney stones.

Lung Cancer

FACTS Lung cancer is on the rise, especially among women. Smoking is responsible for most of the 142,000 deaths due to lung cancer each year, but diet may also play an important role.

Dietary Recommendations

Eat foods rich in beta-carotene (sweet potato, bok choy, winter squash), vitamin C (cantaloupe, strawberries, cranberry juice), vitamin E (wheat germ, broccoli, almonds), folic acid (asparagus, dried beans, sunflower seeds), and vitamin B_6 (fortified cereals, chicken, lean beef).

A major study at Johns Hopkins School of Hygiene and Public Health showed that people who have low blood levels of beta-carotene and vitamin E have a higher rate of lung cancer. Beta-carotene-rich foods include green leafy vegetables (which also contain vitamin E) and yellow and orange fruits and vegetables. Good sources of vitamin E include whole grains, wheat germ, baked sweet potato, almonds, and peanut butter (which is also high in fat, so watch your portion size). Green tea, consumed by the Japanese, has also been shown to have antilung-cancer properties.

Be sure to eat foods rich in Vitamin C—several studies show that people who consume higher levels of vitamin C have lower rates of lung cancer than those who don't. Broccoli, citrus fruits, red pepper, honeydew melon, and asparagus are good C sources.

If you do smoke, keep in mind that smoking depletes your supply of important vitamins and minerals such as beta-carotene, C, E, B_6, and folic acid. Fortified oatmeal and other breakfast cereals are a good source of B_6; folic acid is found in leafy green vegetables such as spinach and broccoli, yeast, wheat germ, and sunflower seeds.

The combination of Vitamin B_{12} and folic acid may help to prevent cancerous changes from occurring in bronchial tissue. If you smoke, talk to your physician about taking a B_{12}/folic acid supplement. I recommend taking 1000 to 2000 mcg B_{12} along with 400 mcg folic acid daily.

Motion Sickness

FACTS Motion sickness or queasiness when traveling in a car (particularly when going up or down hills) or airplane is caused by a disturbance in the inner ear. A 3000-year-old remedy may be the cure!

Dietary Recommendations

Ginger.

Ginger, the common herb used in Chinese medicine, is a potent antinauseant. To make a quick ginger tea, put some sliced, fresh ginger root into a tea ball, place in a teapot, and simmer it in boiling water for ten minutes. A cup or two of this brew will reduce nausea. Ginger root capsules are also available at most natural food stores and are surprisingly effective.

Oral Cancers

FACTS Cancers of the mouth, larynx, and esophagus are closely tied to tobacco use and excess alcohol consumption. Obviously, eliminating these risk factors would go a long way in reducing your risk of developing these forms of cancer. However, diet also plays a role.

Dietary Recommendations

Eat foods rich in vitamin C (mango, honeydew melon, grapefruit) and beta-carotene (papaya, spinach, peach).

Several well-controlled studies showed that a low intake of vitamin C or fruit significantly increased the risk of developing these forms of cancer. Oranges, broccoli, sweet red pepper, strawberries, and watermelon are among the foods that are rich in C. Some studies show that low levels of consumption of fruits and vegetables and low blood levels of beta-carotene have been observed in populations with the highest levels of oral and esophageal cancer. To ensure an adequate supply of beta-carotene, eat green leafy vegetables and yellow and orange fruits and vegetables.

Osteoporosis

FACTS Osteoporosis is caused by the thinning or wearing away of the bones, which can result in a severe loss of bone mass and density, which in turn can make the bones more vulnerable to fractures. Areas that are particularly vulnerable include vertebrae, hip, forearm. About 15 to 20 million Americans have osteoporosis—the majority elderly women—accounting for 1.3 million fractures each year. Osteoporosis tends to strike later in life, when we begin losing more bone than our bodies produce. If you could look at a cross section of bone under a high-powered microscope, you would see that it is actually a spongy protein matrix permeated primarily with calcium and phosphorus salts, with smaller quantities of sodium, magnesium, zinc, iodine, fluoride, and other trace elements. Bone is a hotbed of activity: bone tissue is constantly being formed, broken down, and reformed in a process called remodeling. Osteoclasts are cells that break down bone; osteoblasts are cells that build bone up. During childhood and early adulthood, the osteoblasts (the bone builders) outpace the bone breakers. More bone is created than destroyed, resulting in what we call peak bone mass. Men develop a peak bone mass that is 30 percent more dense than in women, and African-Americans of both sexes develop a bone mass that is roughly 10 percent denser than in whites. Once peak bone mass is reached, at around age 25 or 30, the process levels off, with the amount of bone staying about the same. At around 40, however, the bone breakers outpace the bone builders, and we begin to see a thinning out of the bone, especially in white women. Why does this happen? In the case of women, it appears as if the reduction of estrogen levels, which occurs at around age 40, may make it more difficult for the body to absorb dietary calcium. In addition, several studies suggest that as we age, our bodies are unable to use vitamin D as efficiently, which also affects calcium absorption.

Dietary Recommendations

Eat foods rich in calcium (nonfat dairy products, tofu made with calcium sulfate, canned salmon with bones), vitamin D (fatty fish, fortified milk), boron (prunes, dried fruit), and soy products (tofu, miso soup).

There is some evidence that dietary calcium can retard bone loss. Therefore it is critical for girls and women to eat enough calcium-rich foods. (It's especially important for adolescent girls to get enough calcium while they are developing their peak bone mass.) Unless you are allergic to milk, nonfat milk products are an excellent source of calcium. Nonfat yogurt, which provides nearly 30 percent of the RDA for calcium, is especially gentle on the stomach. In addition, tofu (if made with calcium sulfate), canned salmon and sardines with bones, fortified breakfast cereals (even better with a cup of nonfat milk), and leafy green vegetables such as kale and broccoli are also good sources of calcium.

Vitamin D is essential for the absorption of calcium. Good sources of vitamin D are fortified dairy products and fatty fish.

Another mineral, boron, may also help prevent osteoporosis, by increasing blood estrogen levels. Dried fruits, such as prunes and apricots, are excellent sources of boron.

Soybeans and soybean products, like tofu, are also rich in phytoestrogens, that is, hormonelike substances that mimic estrogen in humans. Some studies suggest that phytoestrogens may relieve some of the more unpleasant symptoms of menopause, and may even protect women from certain forms of cancer. No studies have been done as of yet on whether plant estrogens can help prevent osteoporosis, but as my grandmother used to say about chicken soup, "It can't hurt"—and that was long before researchers discovered that it was potent medicine.

Pancreatic Cancer

FACTS The pancreas is a gland that lies behind the stomach. Cancer of the pancreas is most common in older people; men are slightly more prone than women. Smoking and alcohol consumption increase the odds of getting this form of cancer. At one time, it was believed that coffee was a risk factor for pancreatic cancer; however, recent studies dispute that finding.

Dietary Recommendations

Eat foods rich in lycopene (ruby red grapefruit, red peppers, tomato) and vitamin C (cantaloupe, watermelon, papaya).

Lycopene is a carotenoid that is found in tomatoes, red peppers, and ruby red grapefruits. We know from studies that people who develop pancreatic cancer have lower blood levels of lycopene than those who don't.

Other studies show that people who eat diets rich in vitamin C and fruit (which contains C and lycopene) also have lower rates of pancreatic cancer than people who don't eat such diets.

Although there's no guarantee that vitamin C or lycopene will prevent pancreatic cancer, it certainly makes good sense to include them in your diet.

Prostatic Cancer

FACTS Cancer of the prostate is the most common male cancer in the United States. Some but not all studies suggest that the high-fat American diet may be a contributing factor.

Dietary Recommendations

Eat foods rich in zinc (oysters, wheat germ, pumpkin seed); watch your fat intake.

Men who have a condition known as benign prostatic hypertrophy, or an enlarged prostate—quite common in older men—are at greater risk of developing cancer of the prostate down the road. There are heavy concentrations of zinc in the male prostate, and some nutritionally oriented scientists suspect that a zinc deficiency, which is also quite common in the elderly, may contribute to the onset of prostate problems. I personally think that all men should take a zinc supplement of up to 30 mg daily. In addition, load up on zinc-rich foods, including cooked oysters, lamb chops, brewer's yeast, wheat germ, and pumpkin seeds.

Although the studies on the relationship between dietary fat intake and prostatic cancer have been inconclusive, a high-fat diet is bad for so many other things that it makes good sense to restrict your fat intake anyway.

Psoriasis

FACTS Psoriasis is a common skin disorder, affecting about 1 percent of the population, characterized by the proliferation of cells of the outermost skin layer, which results in red scaly patches on elbows, knees, legs, scalp, and other body parts. The cause of psoriasis is unknown; however, there is a hereditary tendency to develop this disorder. There are several things that can trigger a psoriasis attack, including stress, a throat infection, and rapid weight gain. Although there is no cure, diet and vitamin therapy may help relieve symptoms.

For decades, various diets have been tried on psoriasis patients, to no avail. However, it is generally agreed that a low-fat (especially, low in saturated fat) diet may help to relieve symptoms. In fact, according to one small study, people who ate turkey instead of other meat showed a marked improvement; however, researchers couldn't say whether turkey was actually responsible for the improvement, or whether the real gain came from foregoing other meat, which is high in saturated fat.

Dietary Recommendations

Eat foods rich in omega-3 fatty acids (mackerel, salmon, albacore tuna), vitamin D (fortified milk, fatty fish), psoralens (fruits and vegetables), beta-carotene (sweet potato, spinach, carrots), and selenium (garlic, red grapes, whole grains). Maintain normal weight.

Omega-3 fatty acids, found in fish oil and flaxseed oil, alter the biochemical response in the body that triggers the kind of inflammatory reaction that is believed to bring on psoriasis. Therefore, eating more fatty fish or taking a supplement may help prevent a flare-up.

Fatty fish also contains vitamin D, which is now being used to treat severe cases of psoriasis. For centuries, psoriasis victims have been advised to take sun baths (many use special sunlamps), and indeed, exposure to the sun can often miraculously dry up the angry, red blotches typical of psoriasis. Today, physicians are using a synthetic form of vitamin D to treat psoriasis patients. If you have psoriasis, talk to your physician about this form of therapy. Psoralens, compounds found in vegetables, including celery, parsley, lettuce, limes, and lemons, make the skin more sensitive to sunlight, which may help psoriasis patients. In fact, synthetic psoralens (used externally or orally) may be prescribed to psoriasis patients to enhance the effectiveness of sunlamp treatments.

A sudden weight gain or weight loss may trigger a psoriasis flare-up. Try to maintain normal weight, and if you are dieting, avoid "crash diets"; take off the weight slowly and sensibly.

Bacterial infections, such as strep throat or a yeast infection, may also cause a flare-up. If you have psoriasis, don't let a sore throat or yeast infection go by without seeing your physician. In this case, antibiotics or an antifungal medication may prevent a full-blown psoriasis attack. Also, in keeping with the theme of this book, prevention is the best medicine. Don't allow yourself to get run-down. Eat foods rich in vitamin C, vitamin B_6, vitamin E, and beta-carotene, which will help keep your immune system running at peak efficiency. If you are under a great deal of stress, take a B-complex supplement.

Selenium, found in onion, garlic, chicken, seafood, wheat germ, bran, tuna fish, tomato, and broccoli, may help against the flaky dandruff so prevalent in psoriasis sufferers. If your diet doesn't include these foods, I recommend a supplement of 100 to 200 mcg.

Stomach Cancer

FACTS Refrigeration and better methods of preserving food to prevent bacterial contamination have contributed to a significant drop in stomach cancer in the twentieth century. However, some 24,400 cases of stomach cancer are diagnosed each year, and many could be prevented through proper diet.

Study after study confirms that people who develop stomach cancer eat less fruits and vegetables and have a lower blood level of vitamin C than those who remain cancer-free.

Not coincidentally, most fruits and vegetables are abundant in vitamin C. In addition, several studies show that consumption of dietary fiber was associated with decreased risk of stomach cancer.

Dietary Recommendations

Eat vitamin-C-rich foods (papaya, orange, white potato), berries, fiber, and drink green tea. Avoid smoked, pickled, and cured foods.

Catechins, bioflavonoids found in berries and green tea, may protect against gastrointestinal cancers.

Phenolic acids or phenols, found in garlic, green tea, cereal grains, and cruciferous vegetables (broccoli, cabbage, Brussels sprouts), neutralize nitrosamines, potent carcinogens which are formed in the stomach when nitrates from foods combine with naturally occurring enzymes. In fact, studies in China show that people who eat the most cruciferous vegetables have the lowest levels of stomach cancer, and people who eat the least have the highest levels.

Certain foods are to be avoided. Smoked meats and fish, highly salted foods, and foods with nitrites and nitrates (like bacon and many luncheon meats) also increase your chances of developing stomach cancer. Smoked foods contain potentially carcinogenic tars. Highly salted foods, such as pickled food, also appear to promote cancerous changes in the stomach. Nitrites, which are used to color cured meats, combine with a protein to form nitrosamines; vitamin C helps to deactivate the nitrites and nitrates before they can do their harm.

Stroke

FACTS A stroke will occur when the brain is deprived of oxygen and nutrients due to a rupture or a blockage in a blood vessel. Cerebral thrombosis and cerebral hemorrhages are the most common causes of stroke, and they are caused by blood clots that plug a critical artery feeding the brain. Cigarette smoking, diabetes, high blood pressure, and CAD (coronary artery disease) greatly increase your risk of stroke. Quitting smoking, controlling diabetes, maintaining normal blood pressure, and preventing the formation of plaque in the arteries that can lead to CAD can go a long way in preventing a stroke. In addition, certain foods offer added "stroke protection."

Dietary Recommendations

Eat foods rich in omega-3 fatty acids (sea bass, mackerel, salmon), vitamin E (almond, wheat germ, broccoli), coumarin (found in fruits and vegetables), and selenium (garlic, onion, and broccoli).

Omega-3 fatty acids, found in fatty fish, help to prevent blood clots by lowering blood levels of fibrinogen, a substance that is produced by the body and is necessary for the proper clotting of blood. Too much fibrinogen can promote the formation of blood clots, which can lodge in an artery feeding the brain and cause stroke. Fish such as salmon, mackerel, and sardines are rich in omega-3 fatty acids.

Vitamin E prevents the formation of dangerous blood

clots; good sources include wheat germ, green leafy vegetables, almonds, and vegetable oil.

Coumarins, compounds found in many fruits and vegetables, including parsley, citrus fruits, and cereal grains, are also natural blood thinners.

Garlic contains a substance called ajoene, which also prevents blood clots.

Selenium may also protect against stroke. The states with the lowest selenium levels in their soil have the highest rate of stroke in the United States—the so-called southwestern Stroke Belt. Foods that are rich in selenium include garlic, shellfish, grains, and chicken. A low calcium intake has been linked to strokes as well. (See page 63, calcium.)

Tooth Decay

FACTS Dental caries or cavities are caused by the breakdown of sugar in the mouth which forms an acid that corrodes the tooth enamel. Sugary sweets are a major culprit, but so is any form of carbohydrates, particularly foods that are sticky and actually lodge inside crevices in the teeth. Potato chips, cheese doodles or puffs, and dried fruit are foods that can remain in the mouth for a long time. Proper brushing and flossing can go a long way to eliminate cavities.

Dietary Recommendations

Avoid too many sweets, brush after "sticky" foods, drink green tea, chew on cardamom seed. Possible future remedy: Licorice.

The best way to avoid cavities is to keep your mouth as clean as possible. If you indulge in sweets, brush your teeth immediately after eating them. Avoid sucking candies or chewing gum because the longer the sweet remains in your mouth, the more damage it can cause. (Avoid sugarless gum—it may not cause cavities, but it can cause an upset stomach.) Don't sit around sipping sugary cola drinks or sweetened beverages like coffee or tea: it's equal to giving your mouth a sugar bath.

On the other side of the globe, people have been practicing preventive dentistry for thousands of years. The Japanese typically wash down their desserts with green tea. Researchers recently isolated flavor compounds in Japanese tea that can kill *Streptococcus mutans*, bacteria that may cause the initiation of dental cavities. In India, people traditionally end their meals with bowls of spices, including cardamom seed, which people there have been chewing for thousands of years. Recently, a University of California, Berkeley, chemist who investigated cardamom for potential medicinal properties discovered that it contained ingredients that had antibiotic action against bacteria that promote cavities. Be on the look out for cardamom-flavored toothpastes and mouthwashes!

In the not too distant future, a form of licorice also may be marketed as a means of preventing cavities. Glycyrrhizin, a compound found in licorice root, has been shown to retard tooth decay. Unfortunately, you will not get the same benefit from the licorice-flavored candy on the market in the United States; it contains little licorice, and is often flavored with anise. However, in Europe, licorice root candy is already being marketed as a tooth saver, in addition to its other potential benefits (it's a cancer fighter and an anti-inflammatory).

CAUTION Licorice should be avoided by people who have high blood pressure or heart problems since it depletes the body of potassium.

Xerophthalmia (Night Blindness)

FACTS In xerophthalmia, the cornea and conjunctiva become dried out and wrinkled. It is caused by a vitamin A deficiency, and can lead to night blindness.

Dietary Recommendations

Eat foods rich in beta-carotene (yellow and orange vegetables and fruits and dark leafy green vegetables).

Vitamin A combines with a protein in the eye to form visual purple, the substance that enables us to see in the dark. Therefore, in order to keep your vision sharp, day or night, eat lots of beta-carotene-rich foods, such as apricots, broccoli, sweet potatoes, mango, pumpkin, and yellow squash. (Beta-carotene is converted into vitamin A as the body needs it.)

Yeast Infection (Monilial Infection)

FACTS Monilial infections, which often strike women, are caused by a yeastlike fungus, *Candida albicans,* that normally lives in the mouth, vaginal and intestinal tract. Certain situations can throw off the balance beween good and bad bacteria in the body, which can result in an overgrowth of *Candida*. The result: an itchy, uncomfortable discharge. About one out of ten women have recurrent monilial infections. Thrush, an infection of the mouth that is also caused by *Candida*, often strikes AIDS patients and other people with compromised immune systems.

Dietary Recommendations

Eat yogurt and immune-boosting foods (garlic, shiitake mushrooms).

Yogurt has been a longtime folk remedy for yeast infection. It took a woman physician from Long Island, New York, to do a serious investigation of whether yogurt works. Based on her findings, it does. In her study, women who ate 8 ounces of yogurt each day for six months had significantly fewer yeast infections than those who did not. Not every brand of yogurt will be effective against *Candida:* the yogurt must contain active cultures of *Lactobacillus acidophilus*. Will yogurt work as well in preventing thrush in AIDS patients? As far as I know, no one has done any serious studies on this; however, it just might help.

In addition, anyone who is plagued with chronic candidal infection needs to keep the immune system working well. Immune boosters such as garlic and shiitake mushrooms may help strengthen your ability to fight against infection.

CHAPTER 7

A Woman's Body

I devote a good deal of time to traveling around the country, lecturing on nutrition and appearing on talk shows. Within the past year or two, I've noticed an interesting trend: Women, who used to typically ask questions about their husband's or their children's health, are now becoming very concerned about their own health. I consider this to be a very healthy sign.

With breast cancer on the rise, and the growing awareness of heart disease as a problem that affects women as well as men, women need to be vigilant about protecting their own health.

Here are some of the most important questions that women commonly ask me about nutrition and/or supplements.

I'm in my late forties and three of my friends have already had mastectomies and, frankly, I'm frightened. What can I do to protect myself against breast cancer?

It is frightening that one out of nine American women will eventually get breast cancer. Although we don't know for sure how to prevent this disease, or even what causes it, researchers are beginning to unravel the mystery of breast cancer. Several studies have shown that women who eat fruits and vegetables rich in beta-carotene and vitamin C have lower levels of breast cancer. Eating your five fruits and vegetables daily, and perhaps taking a beta-carotene supplement (10,000 IU daily) and a vitamin C supplement (1000 mg daily), may make a difference in whether you develop this or any other form of cancer.

Selenium may also protect against breast cancer. I recommend that you take a supplement of 100 mcg daily. Good food sources of selenium include garlic, shellfish, wheat germ, grains, tuna fish, and chicken.

We also know that women who get breast cancer tend to have higher blood levels of estrogen than women who don't; estrogen can promote the growth of mammary tumors. There is some evidence that women who eat a diet high in certain types of fiber may have lower estrogen levels than those who don't. A recent study sponsored by the American Health Foundation actually measured the estrogen levels in premenopausal women who were given 15 to 30 grams of wheat, corn, or oat bran. After two months, women on wheat bran showed a dramatic drop in estrogens, but not the women on corn or oat bran.

Several studies have shown that broccoli and other members of the cabbage family contain many compounds that can deactivate potent estrogens. In addition, soy products such as tofu or miso may also help reduce blood estrogen levels (women who are salt-sensitive, however, should avoid soy, since it is high in sodium). To sum up:

Earl Mindell's Daily Anti-Breast-Cancer Regimen

15 grams of wheat bran* (equivalent to 1 tablespoon)
1 cup serving of either broccoli, cabbage, Brussels sprouts, or bok choy

2 servings of fruits or vegetables high in beta-carotene
2 servings of fruits or vegetables high in vitamin C
½ cup serving of tofu, soybeans†

* If you're not used to eating bran, begin slowly, gradually increasing your
  intake.
† Soybeans and soy sauce are usually high in sodium; avoid these foods if
  you have high blood pressure.

Last, but definitely not least, diet alone cannot protect you against breast cancer. Women should examine their breasts monthly for signs of irregularity, and women over 50 should talk to their physicians about an annual mammogram.

> *Help! My mother had a bad case of osteoporosis and I don't want to end up like she did. She never took care of herself; she smoked, ate poorly, and never exercised. I'm 45: What should I be doing right now to avoid getting "bent out of shape"?*

The tendency to develop osteoporosis can be hereditary, but your mother's fate is not necessarily your own. Sedentary women who smoke are at higher risk of developing this disease than nonsmoking women who are active. In fact, several studies have shown that exercise, such as walking or mild weight lifting can help to maintain bone mass in women. (Check with your physician before embarking on an exercise program.)

In addition, diet may also play a role. Until very recently, researchers disagreed about whether increased calcium could slow bone loss after menopause. An important New Zealand study published in the *New England Journal of Medicine* reported that women who took 1000 mg of calcium in addition to what they were getting in their food reduced their bone loss by one third to one half. These women were getting about 750 mg of calcium in their diets, which incidentally is more than American women typically consume, but less than the recommended amount for women their age. (Many experts now recommend that postmenopausal women consume between 1200 to 1500 mg of calcium daily.) If you decide to take a calcium supplement, you should also take up to 400 to 800 IU of vitamin D to increase absorption. Watch your caffeine and alcohol intake; both are calcium zappers. In addition, go light on the salt; sodium may promote the excretion of calcium in the urine. Avoid foods that are high in oxalic acid (chocolate, spinach, and Swiss chard), which can also interfere with calcium absorption.

I just found out that I was pregnant, and I'm thrilled. I'm not thrilled by the fact that my physician just handed me a prescription for prenatal vitamins without telling me anything else about nutrition. What do I need to know?

Popping a vitamin pill is not enough to ensure a healthy pregnancy. First, you need to eat a good well-balanced diet. On average, a normal-weight pregnant woman needs to consume around 300 additional calories in her daily diet to ensure that the new life will get adequate nourishment. Eating less may result in a low-birth-weight baby, who may not be as hardy as a normal-weight one.

Being pregnant, however, is not a license to gorge. Excess weight can also be dangerous. Loading up on high-fat junk food, especially early in the pregnancy, may put on weight too quickly. Later, just when your developing baby needs good nutrition, you may have to cut back on food.

Pregnant women must be vigilant about getting enough vitamins and minerals. Calcium, which is usually lacking from a woman's diet, is extremely important during pregnancy—you will need to make sure that you are getting your full 1200 mg daily. Most prenatal vitamins have only 15 to 25 percent of the RDA for this mineral, so you must add more calcium-rich foods to your diet. If you don't, the baby may sap your calcium stores, which could result in osteoporosis. Calcium may also help prevent preeclampsia, a very dangerous complication of pregnancy, by keeping blood pressure within normal levels. In addition, leg cramps, the bane of pregnancy, can often be alleviated by adding extra calcium to your diet. Nonfat or low-fat dairy products are your best sources of calcium. Eat at least one carton of low-fat or nonfat yogurt daily: it not only provides a calcium boost, but protects against vaginal yeast infections, which are quite common during pregnancy.

Folic acid is also critical for the prevention of birth defects, especially in the first month after conception. Although your prenatal prescription vitamin includes the RDA for folic acid, I still suggest that you eat foods rich in this important B vitamin. Good sources include liver, whole grains, dark green leafy vegetables, eggs, and orange juice. Women who have been taking oral contraceptives may have lower stores of folic acid, and therefore should talk to their physician about taking a supplement, preferably before they even get pregnant.

Vitamin C is also important for mothers-to-be and their babies. A recent study has shown that cancerous brain tumors are more common in children whose mothers had a low level of this vitamin during pregnancy. Eat lots of fruits and vegetables, including sweet red peppers, oranges, mangoes, watermelon, and broccoli. (This will also help prevent another common malady of pregnancy—constipation.)

Also keep in mind that you will need more iron, copper,

and zinc. Iron is essential for the formation of red blood cells. If the expectant mother is short on this mineral, she could become anemic. Copper and zinc help the body fight off infection; low levels of these minerals may contribute to complications such as premature birth.

Make sure that your diet is rich in antioxidants—beta-carotene, vitamins C and E, and selenium. A recent study done at the University of Cincinnati suggests that women with preeclampsia had only half as much antioxidant activity in their blood as women who do not get this disorder. This doesn't mean that antioxidants can prevent preeclampsia, but it does suggest that they have a role to play in keeping women healthy during pregnancy.

Avoid drinking alcoholic beverages; alcohol can cause fetal alcohol syndrome, a severe form of retardation. At one time, it was believed that caffeine in coffee could cause birth defects, but recent studies show that coffee in moderate amounts (1 to 2 cups daily) is all right.

Earl Mindell's Recipe for Morning Sickness

To alleviate nausea and discomfort caused by hormonal changes, drink a cup of ginger root tea or take a ginger root tablet or capsule first thing in the morning. Throughout the day, sip ginger ale or peppermint tea.

Around ten days before my period, I begin to feel bloated and irritable. My breasts get tender, and sometimes I get a headache right before I begin to menstruate. Any advice?

About half of all premenopausal women experience some form of premenstrual syndrome (PMS), which includes the types of symptoms that you are describing—excessive water retention, mood swings, and a general feeling of discomfort. There are things that you can do to lessen the severity of PMS. First, avoid salty foods that promote fluid retention and eat natural diuretics that promote excretion. (Good natural diuretics include asparagus, celery, dandelion leaves, and carrot.) Second, many women with PMS also find that caffeine aggravates their symptoms; therefore drink decaffeinated coffee, herbal teas, and other no-caffeine beverages.

In addition, get more calcium into your life. A recent study of a small group of women showed that nearly all the women who complained of PMS had less severe and fewer symptoms after consuming a high-calcium diet (1200 mg daily).

Finally, you might consider taking evening primrose oil, which comes in capsules. Several studies in England and Canada have shown that women with severe PMS were greatly helped by this natural remedy. For best results, take three (250 mg each) capsules daily, starting around mid-cycle until menstruation begins.

I'm on birth control pills, and I want to know if The Pill affects my nutritional needs.

It certainly does! First, oral contraceptives sap the body of important B vitamins—B_6, B_{12}, and folic acid—and vitamin C. Increase your intake of food rich in these vitamins; depending on your diet, you may need to take a supplement. Avoid drinking too much alcohol; it depletes the body of B-complex vitamins, which you're losing already.

Any woman on The Pill also needs to watch her blood lipid levels very carefully. Most birth control pills are a combination of estrogen and progesterone. Estrogen raises triglyceride levels, which may increase the risk of heart disease in some women. Progesterone raises LDL, the bad cholesterol, and decreases the beneficial HDL, which increases your risk of developing coronary artery disease. After you go on The Pill, your physician should monitor your blood lipid levels very carefully. If they go into the danger zone, your physician may try switching pills—different forms of progesterone may affect different women in different ways—or putting you on a different form of contraception. If you're on a high-fat diet, switching to a low-fat diet may help to maintain normal cholesterol and triglyceride levels. In addition, increasing your antioxidant vitamins and minerals (beta-carotene, C, E, and selenium) may help to keep your LDL cholesterol in check.

I'm in my early fifties and have just become menopausal. Frankly, I'm being driven crazy by hot flashes and vaginal dryness, which I know are normal but are certainly uncomfortable. My physician suggested that I try estrogen replacement therapy, but it goes against my grain to treat menopause like an illness that needs to be "treated" with a pill. Are there any natural solutions to my problems?

Your concerns are shared by many women: in fact, I get asked more questions about menopause these days than any other topic. Like you, many women bristle at the notion of being treated by a drug. Menopause is not an illness; it is a natural part of life. A dip in estrogen levels causes many of the symptoms that women like least, such as hot flashes and vaginal dryness, headaches, fatigue, depression, and insomnia. In addition, after menopause, women are more prone to develop osteoporosis and heart disease. Some women may breeze through menopause easily. Others, like yourself, may not feel quite up to par.

Interestingly enough, in Japan and some other Oriental countries, women rarely complain about menopausal symptoms. In fact, there's no word for menopause in Japanese! Some experts contend that women may actually have these symptoms but, in keeping with Oriental stoicism, just don't complain. However, I think that Japanese women may actually feel better because of their diets. The Japanese diet is rich in soy products (miso, tofu, soybeans) which are abundant in phytoestrogens, hormonelike compounds that mimic the action of estrogen in humans. As natural estrogen levels begin to drop, these plant estrogens may take their place. Chinese women rely on an herb, dong quai, also high in phytoestrogens, to control the discomfort of menopause. Throughout the Orient, women sip ginseng tea, another rich source of plant estrogens.

Many American women swear that their hot flashes are controlled by vitamin E supplements (400 IU mixed tocopherols). In addition, I often recommend a good B-complex supplement for women who complain of depression.

Increasing your calcium intake (1500 mg daily) and watching your fat intake will help keep you healthy throughout menopause.

I'm in my sixties and have just begun a walking program. Do I need any extra vitamins or minerals?

First, let me congratulate you. Your walking program will help prevent heart disease and osteoporosis, two diseases that are prevalent among women in your age group. I guarantee that you will also look and feel better.

Exercise will increase your need for riboflavin, Vitamin B_2, which is found in milk, cheese, yogurt, beef, fortified breads and cereal, and vegetables including broccoli. A recent study showed that older women who exercise need additional riboflavin to maintain normal blood levels. Eat plenty of complex carbohydrates—whole grains, legumes, fruit and vegetables—to provide the fuel for your walk. Also, don't forget the most important food supplement of all—water. As you sweat, your need for water increases. Drink at least 6 to 8 glasses a day; bring a water bottle along for extra long walks, or if it's a hot day.

I used to worry that my husband would be the one in my family to have a heart attack, but now I'm worried about me. My physician told me that although my cholesterol is on the high end of normal, I have very high triglycerides (300 mg/dl) and low HDLs, which means that I'm at added risk of having a heart attack. I'm overweight and I'm not too careful about what I eat. To add to my bad profile, I've just become menopausal. What can I do to prevent heart disease?

You're right to be concerned. A woman's risk of having a heart attack greatly increases after menopause. However, there are things that you can do to improve your chances of remaining heart-attack-free.

First, you have to start being careful about what you eat. You need to eat a low-fat diet, very low in saturated fat and high in complex carbohydrates and fiber. Fruits and vegetables are in; steaks and cheeseburgers are out. Keep total fat intake to under 25 percent of your daily calories, with saturated fat under 10 percent. Olive oil, a monounsaturated fat, can help increase your HDLs, but use it sparingly. Two to 3 teaspoons a day in your cooking or salad dressing is enough to gain maximum benefit. A regular exercise program will also help raise your HDLs. Some people may advise you to drink a glass of red wine daily, which also can increase HDLs. However, in your case, that would not be wise because wine also increases triglycerides. You may be able to get the same benefit without the liability by eating red grapes or drinking Concord grape juice.

Omega-3 fatty acids, found in fish, are good triglyceride busters. (You need to reduce your triglyceride level to under 190.) Eat between two and three fatty fish meals a week. Chili peppers have also been shown to reduce triglycerides as well as cholesterol.

Finally, make sure that you're getting enough antioxidants, which can prevent plaque formation in arteries. Eat foods high in vitamins C and E, beta-carotene, and selenium.

If diet alone doesn't work, talk to your physician about taking a combination niacin/chromium supplement, which can also cut cholesterol and triglycerides.

After my baby was born, people advised me to breast-feed so that I would lose weight faster. Since the birth of my baby, I haven't lost any significant amount of weight—in fact, I may have gained a few pounds. Where did I go wrong?

The only thing wrong is your expectation that you would lose weight faster by breast-feeding. In fact, a recent study shows that just the opposite may be true—women who don't breast-feed may take off weight faster than those who do. Researchers aren't sure why this is the case; however, they suspect that breast-feeding moms may still be eating for two, and that women who no longer breast-feed may face up to the fact earlier that, in order to lose weight, they're going to have to cut back on calories and increase exercise.

CHAPTER 8

A Man's Body

The following are questions that men commonly ask about nutrition and vitamin/mineral supplements.

> *I just turned 50 and my internist suggested that I have a transrectal ultrasound exam—a fairly new diagnostic test—to screen early prostate cancer. At first, I thought that he was being alarmist, but when he told me how common this form of cancer is, I began to worry. What should I be doing to protect myself?*

The statistics are frightening—14 percent of all men over 50 will get prostate cancer. In fact, it is the second most common cancer among men (skin cancer tops the list). African-American men are at a slightly greater risk than Caucasian men, but this is one problem that every male needs to be concerned about. Although we don't know what causes prostate cancer, there are some measures that you can take that may tip the scales in your favor.

First, several studies worldwide have shown a correlation between cancer of the prostate and a high-fat diet. Japanese men who live in Hawaii—who presumably are eating the standard high-fat American fare—have a significantly higher rate of prostate cancer than those who live in Japan, where they are eating the traditional low-fat Japanese diet. Even if seaweed and sushi are not exactly your favorite foods, you may reduce your risk of prostate cancer by cutting your daily fat intake to under 20 percent of your total calories. (The average American diet is about 40 percent fat.)

We also know that men who get prostate cancer have lower blood levels of two crucial minerals: selenium and zinc. Selenium is an antioxidant that helps protect cells from the kind of damage that could initiate the growth of cancerous tumors. Men in particular need this mineral—almost half of their body's supply is concentrated in the testicles and portions of the seminal ducts adjacent to the prostate gland. People who live in areas where the soil is rich in this mineral tend to have lower rates of cancer. Good sources of selenium include garlic, shellfish, grains, and chicken. If you live in a selenium-poor area, consider taking a supplement. Selenium can be toxic in very high doses, so do not exceed 200 mcg daily.

Zinc is another mineral that is heavily concentrated in the male prostate. Zinc is believed to regulate the metabolism of testosterone in the prostate, and there is some evidence that an imbalance of testosterone may contribute to the growth of tumors in the prostate. Zinc is abundant in oysters, lamb chops, and wheat germ.

Foods that regulate hormones may play a role in helping to prevent hormone-dependent cancers such as prostatic cancer. Studies of Japanese men and women reveal low rates of breast cancer and prostatic cancer, two very different diseases that have one common link: Hormones (estrogen for women, and testosterone for men) can trigger tumor growth in the breast and prostate. Japanese men and women have yet another common ground—their diet is rich in soybean products, which are high in phytochemicals that are converted to biologically active hormonelike substances in the intestine. These plant-derived "hormones" may deactivate potent hormones in the body that can initiate the growth of cancerous tumors on certain sites. Soybeans and soy-based foods such as tofu and miso may offer some protection against prostatic cancer.

My wife and I are planning on starting a family. Her physician put her on a vitamin supplement; is there anything that I should be taking to ensure that we conceive a healthy baby?

Vitamin C and zinc. Researcher Bruce Ames of the University of California at Berkeley conducted a small study involving ten men in which he examined the quality of sperm produced by the men on a vitamin-C-deficient diet (5 mg daily), compared with the same men on a vitamin-C-supplemented diet (up 250 mg daily). The men on the C-deficient diet showed increased levels of DNA damage in their sperm—the kind of damage that may be responsible for birth defects in their offspring. DNA damage declined only when the men were given the RDA of 60 mg of vitamin C or more daily. If you're planning on conceiving a child, eat foods rich in vitamin C and/or take a supplement.

Zinc is also essential for the success of your endeavor. A zinc deficiency can lead to a low sperm count, a leading cause of infertility in men. Eat plenty of oysters and wheat germ and munch on pumpkin seeds to keep your zinc supply replenished.

Finally, if you smoke, quit before you conceive. At least two studies have shown that children of men who smoke have higher rates of leukemia and lymphoma than children of nonsmoking fathers. (Smoking zaps vitamin C from your system, which is why the RDA for smokers is 100 mg.)

*I'm a graduate student who works long hours and has
poor eating habits. I don't take vitamins, and my day
often ends scarfing down a burger and fries at the
local fast-food restaurant so I can get back to the
library. The problem is, I recently married an attorney
who also works long hours. Frankly, by the time my
wife and I are together at night, I'm too exhausted—
and not exactly overly interested—in sex. Help! This
is no way to build an enduring relationship.*

Let me assure you that you are not alone. Because of our
hectic life-styles, especially among working couples, many
of the men and women I speak with complain about fatigue
and lack of sex drive. Although there is no magic potion or
aphrodisiac that can get your juices flowing again, there are
things that you can do to rekindle your sex life.

First, cut out those burgers and fries. A recent study
showed that fatty food can actually reduce the production
of testosterone, the male sex hormone that regulates sex
drive. However, low-fat food does not adversely affect testosterone, so load up on more grains, fresh fruits and vegetables. Stick to lean cuts of meat, skinless poultry, and
broiled fish. If you don't have time to cook, find a diner or a
family-style restaurant that offers a few low-fat entrées.

Eat foods rich in zinc, which is essential for a healthy
male reproductive system. Oysters, wheat germ, yeast, and
pumpkin seeds are good choices.

In addition, to counteract the stress in your life, I would
recommend a special stress-formulated B-complex supplement. Finally, a moderate exercise program—a brisk walk
for a half hour daily or a lunchtime swim at the school
gym—may do wonders for your evening stamina. (For

more information, read Earl Mindell's Super Sexy Diet at
the end of this chapter.)

*All through my teens, I worked as a lifeguard at my
local pool, where my main concern was getting as tan
as I could. Today, I work as a high school football
coach, where I am also constantly exposed to the
outdoors. I know better now, and I try to wear
sunscreen to avoid burning. Is there anything else
I can do to avoid skin cancer?*

Good question—skin cancer is the most common cancer
to afflict men. First, I hope that you and your physician carefully check for any changes in your skin that could signal a
problem. Early detection is essential for effective treatment.

Second, in addition to eating foods rich in beta-carotene
(yellow and orange fruits and vegetables and green leafy vegetables), you should take a beta-carotene supplement—
10,000 IU should do it. Beta-carotene converts to vitamin
A as your body needs it. Derivatives of vitamin A and other
members of the retinoid family are used as treatments for
certain forms of skin cancer.

Third, I would recommend eating a diet rich in antioxidants (beta-carotene, vitamins C and E, and selenium).
There is strong evidence that antioxidants may prevent the
abnormal changes in cells that can lead to conditions such
as skin cancer.

Finally, cover up when you go into the sun, especially
between the hours of 10 A.M. and 2 P.M. when the rays are
the strongest. Be sure to wear sunscreen (I recommend SPF
of 15 or above), a shirt, and a hat as added protection for
your face. Sunglasses are also important as overexposure to
ultraviolet rays can cause cataracts.

*I'm on a weight-loss diet and have recently begun
working out at the gym. What should I be eating to
improve my performance? (P.S. What can I do to
alleviate post-workout soreness?)*

To answer your first question, if you're on a low-calorie
diet, you may not be getting enough nutrients to support
your workout. You may need to supplement your food with
additional beta-carotene, B-complex, C, E, iron, and zinc.

Before working out, stick to high-energy foods such as
whole grains, pasta with a low-fat sauce, fruit salad, yogurt,
and other complex carbohydrates that will burn slowly, providing you with the fuel to keep going. (Eat at least one to
two hours before working out to give yourself enough time
to digest your food.) Avoid sugary foods like candy bars that
provide a quick charge, and then leave you feeling tired and
let down.

Now, about those aching muscles. Recently, researchers
at Tufts University found that the muscle soreness that
occurs after working out may be caused by oxidative damage due to the stress of exercise. They found that taking a
vitamin E supplement daily may improve athletic stamina
as well as reducing the postexercise muscle soreness. Between
400 and 800 IU of vitamin E daily (depending on your
food intake of vitamin E) may make waking up the day after
a workout a bit easier.

*I'm a chemist and I know that my risk of developing
certain forms of cancer is higher than for nonchemists.
I love my job, but would like to do all I can to reduce
my risk of cancer. Any advice?*

Exposure to carcinogens in the workplace accounts for
about 10 percent of all cancers. Chemists in particular have

somewhat higher rates of brain cancer, lymphoma, leukemia, and pancreatic cancer. Other occupations have their own particular risk factors depending on the carcinogens that are commonly used. Since you are aware of these problems, I assume that you are doing everything that you're supposed to do at the work site in terms of safety. Even though they are time-consuming and may seem a bit bothersome, safety regulations are for your protection. Be scrupulous about following them! There are some other things that you can do to protect yourself further.

Make sure that your workplace is well ventilated and preferably smoke-free. Cigarette smoking and exposure to known carcinogens such as asbestos can greatly increase your risk of cancer.

Diet may also play a major role in preventing carcinogens from doing you any harm. Try to eat a lot of "detoxifiers," that is, foods that may thwart the initiation or growth of cancer. Foods rich in beta-carotene, selenium, and vitamins C and E are among your best choices. Cook with garlic, munch on parsley, load up on broccoli and bok choy. Begin the day with half a cantaloupe. Eat lots of citrus fruit, which contains terpenes, compounds that help the body to fight off carcinogens. Make sure that you're getting enough fiber, which also helps to rid the body of toxins. Avoid eating too much fat—toxins are stored in fatty tissue in the body.

Even if you do everything right, there is a chance that you will still get cancer. However, I believe that by paying close attention to nutrition, you are greatly improving your odds of staying well.

I'm only 35 and I'm beginning to lose my hair! I don't take any vitamins and I usually eat whatever I can on the run. If I reform my ways, can I save my hair?

I wish I could tell you that there was a tried and true way to prevent baldness, but there isn't. Hair loss is largely determined by genetics. Although there are few legitimate treatments, some people have had success with the drug minoxidil. Talk to your physician to see if you are a good candidate. However, a sluggish thyroid or other medical problem may also trigger hair loss, and once treated, the condition often reverses itself. In other cases, a severe vitamin or mineral deficiency may cause baldness; however, that kind of deficiency is rare.

Although there is no guarantee that switching to a healthier diet and increasing the amount of vitamins in your life will prevent hair loss, it will at least help keep the bounce and shine in the hair that you've got left. Eat lots of foods rich in the B vitamin biotin, which include brewer's yeast, raw or roasted nuts, and whole grain foods. Biotin deficiency in animals can cause hair loss. Another member of the B family, inositol, may also help maintain healthy hair: It is found in cantaloupe, liver, brewer's yeast, cabbage, lima beans, and wheat germ. In addition, make sure that you are getting enough vitamin C and folic acid.

My Chinese friends swear that fo-ti, sold in most health food stores today, will prevent hair from going gray and other signs of premature aging.

Earl Mindell's Super Sexy Diet

Good nutrition and great sex go hand in hand. Here's some advice on what to eat to feel healthy and sexy.

- Eat lots of green, yellow, and orange vegetables and fruits rich in beta-carotene. The body converts beta-carotene into vitamin A according to your needs. Vitamin A is essential in the production of all sex hormones. (In women, vitamin A counteracts the negative effect of estrogen, which, if supplied in excess, reduces your sexual desire.)

- Nuts, whole grains (7 to 10 servings of grains, breads, and cereals daily), dried beans, peas, and beets are a must because they contain manganese, a mineral that assists in the production of dopamine, a neurotransmitter (sends impulses from the blood to the brain) that tends to heighten or "turn on" your sexual arousal.

- Bone up on B_6 (found in whole grains, liver, kidney, fish, yeast, avocados, soybeans, cantaloupe, black-strap molasses, unmilled rice, eggs, oats, peanuts, and walnuts). B_6 decreases prolactin, a hormone that can diminish a woman's sexual desire. It also increases the hormone in men that regulates testosterone, which maintains male sexual characteristics.

- Swing with zinc (found in oysters, wheat germ, cashews, lean beef, lamb, lean pork, green beans, lima beans, pumpkin seeds, nonfat milk, and ground mustard). These zinc-rich foods stimulate the formation of testosterone, therefore aiding a man's ability for erections and ejaculation.

- E is for everybody. Chow down on green vegetables, whole grains, wheat germ, nuts, seeds, soybeans, Brussels sprouts, and spinach. Add unrefined vegetable oils and whole grain cereals to your daily diet. Vitamin E, an anticoagulant (blood thinner), improves circulation throughout your body, including to your sexual organs. It also aids in the production of prostaglandins, fatty acids that cause contractions of the uterus during intercourse.

◆ If all else fails, look for my book *Earl Mindell's Herb Bible*. In it I discuss yohimbe, an herb that is the only known aphrodisiac. It's available in prescription strength from your physician and should be used only under a doctor's supervision.

CHAPTER 9

Foods for Special Needs

Nutritional needs vary from person to person, depending on life-style and general health. The following section answers some of the types of questions that I am routinely asked about specific problems.

I'm a smoker who is currently in between smoking cessation programs. I know I have to stop, but it's really hard. Until I can kick the habit, are there any foods that I should be eating that can alleviate the bad health effects of smoking?

Before I begin, let me caution you that there are no vitamin pills or so-called power foods that can undo the harm that you are inflicting upon yourself every time you light up. However, there are some things that you can do that may somewhat reduce your risk of developing a smoking-related disorder. First, smoking saps the body of vitamin C, which protects against cancer and heart disease—as a smoker you are at greater risk of developing either of these potentially deadly illnesses. Every cigarette you smoke destroys between 25 to 100 mg of this critical vitamin. To avoid falling short of C, eat a vitamin-C-rich fruit or vegetable for every cigarette you smoke. Think of it this way: 1 orange (70 mg of vitamin C) = 1 cigarette; 1 sweet red pepper (180 mg of vitamin C) = 2 cigarettes. You'll be so busy munching, you may actually cut down on your smoking! By the way, strawberries are a particularly good food choice for smokers. Not only are they packed with vitamin C, but they are rich in ellagic acid, which has been shown to destroy hydrocarbons, potentially carcinogenic compounds found in tobacco smoke that can wreak havoc on your lungs.

Second, eat foods rich in beta-carotene. Some studies suggest that beta-carotene may offer some protection against cancer for smokers. Many foods with vitamin C, such as broccoli and mango, offer a good amount of beta-carotene, and may also contain cancer-fighting compounds. Watch your alcohol intake; for many people, heavy alcohol consumption and smoking are a deadly combination. In addition, you should make sure that you're getting enough of antioxidants E and selenium, which may help prevent the initiation of cancerous changes in cells.

At least one study reported in the *American Journal of Clinical Nutrition* noted that vitamin B_{12} and folic acid may reduce the cancer risk for male smokers (and possibly for women, too, although the study was performed on male subjects). Male smokers with potentially cancerous changes in their bronchial tubes were given a B_{12} and folic acid supplement. Those on the supplement developed fewer dangerous cells than male smokers not on the supplement. I recommend 1000 to 2000 mcg daily sublingual B_{12} with 400 mcg folic acid. If you use the nasal gel form of B_{12}, take 400 mcg of B_{12} nasal gel every second or third day, along with 400 mcg folic acid daily.

Finally, keep your other risk factors for heart disease in check: don't allow your blood cholesterol or triglycerides to reach unhealthy levels. Make sure your blood pressure is normal. Try to get enough exercise without overexerting yourself (neither your heart nor your lungs should be put under too much strain).

I have a hunch that once you begin taking care of yourself, you will be all the more motivated to break this deadly habit.

Every time I drink a glass of milk or indulge in an ice cream cone, I get diarrhea and a stomachache. My doctor said that I must be milk-intolerant and suggested that I simply lay off dairy products. The only problem is, my gynecologist told me that I was prone to osteoporosis and suggested that I eat a lot of milk products. What should I do?

Milk intolerance is a very common problem that affects millions of adults, especially those of African and southern European descent. The problem is caused by lactose, a milk sugar in dairy products that is digested by an enzyme in the small intestine called lactase. People who are lactose-intolerant do not produce enough lactase; therefore, they have difficulty digesting dairy foods.

You have several options. First, dairy products are not the only source of calcium: Other good sources include tofu made with calcium sulfate, canned salmon or sardines with bones, and leafy green vegetables such as kale. However, it may be more difficult to get your full RDA of calcium from these foods. For example, it would take three cups of cooked kale to equal the amount of calcium in one glass of milk. In addition, the calcium in dairy products is more easily absorbed by the body than calcium from other sources.

Some lactose-intolerant people have no difficulty digesting

yogurt if it has active cultures and if it is true yogurt—not the highly sugared, parfait-style stuff that often passes for yogurt. You can find real yogurt in many health food stores, or you can make your own.

In addition, there are special lactose-free dairy products on the market that are sold in many supermarkets. Check in your local dairy case. If you can't find them in your neighborhood, keep in mind that these products are often sold in markets that cater to an older or ethnic population.

You can also try a lactase-enzyme supplement which helps to digest the lactose in dairy foods. Some supplements come in liquid form that can be mixed right into milk; others must be taken during or right after eating a dairy food.

> *I have to travel a lot on my job, especially to Mexico and the Caribbean. Most people would be thrilled with these kinds of assignments, but not me. After two or three days on the road, I suffer from an upset stomach and diarrhea. What can I do?*

Changes in soil content, water, and sanitation procedures contribute to "traveler's diarrhea." My first and most obvious advice is to watch what you eat and drink. Steer clear of raw fruits and vegetables—never eat any fruit or vegetable that hasn't been peeled. If you order bottled water, make sure it is served to you in a sealed bottle: all too often, in many hotels, bottles are filled directly from the tap. (I've seen this done myself many times.) Also, pass on the ice cubes—you can't be sure what kind of water they're made of.

I have also found taking an acidophilus supplement (3 capsules or 2 tablespoons of liquid daily) can help ward off diarrhea by maintaining the proper balance of good and bad bacteria in the intestine. Be sure to eat lots of yogurt with active cultures before your trip and lots of yogurt on your return.

I do a lot of business entertaining, and although the three-martini lunch is no longer in vogue, I've found that during some hectic weeks, I still drink one to two glasses of wine or a mixed drink (like a piña colada) daily. Do I need any special foods or supplements?

First, I want to caution you that alcohol can be very fattening. The average glass of wine weighs in at about 90 calories; your piña colada is well over 250 calories. Alcohol also slows down your metabolism, making it more difficult for your body to burn fat. If you find that your waistline is expanding, consider cutting back on your drinking, or switching to mineral water with a twist. You can also water down your wine with seltzer or club soda (or order a spritzer) and nurse your drink carefully throughout lunch or dinner.

Second, alcohol can interfere with the absorption of some very important vitamins. B-complex vitamins in particular are vulnerable to alcohol; therefore, be sure to take a supplement as well as eat foods rich in these vitamins. Finally, alcohol also hampers the absorption of vitamin C, so increase your intake. One easy way to replenish your C is to drink a glass of orange, tomato or pineapple juice instead of an alcoholic beverage.

If I don't have my morning cup of coffee, I get a horrible headache. In fact, sometimes I need several cups to get me started, and by midafternoon I need several cups more, but if I drink coffee in the afternoon, I have trouble falling asleep. But if I don't, I'm ready to fall asleep at the office. How can I get off this vicious cycle?

When you're on the caffeine roller coaster, it can be hard to get off. In fact, a recent study showed that people who drink far less coffee than you can also become "caffeine-dependent." Even a one or two cup a day person may experience withdrawal symptoms such as a headache, nausea, and excessive fatigue if he or she tries to go cold turkey.

In your case, I have a hunch that too much caffeine may be causing your afternoon drowsiness. Caffeine provides its lift by stimulating the release of stored sugar from the liver. It's effect, however, is short-acting. After the initial boost, many people experience fatigue as the effects of the caffeine wear off. In addition, excessive caffeine can cause nervousness, irritability, and insomnia, as well as other problems. Caffeine also saps the body of important vitamins and minerals, including B-complex (especially thiamine), zinc, vitamin C, and potassium. When "caffeine addicts" finally cut back on coffee, they find that they have a lot more energy, and I think that you will, too.

Tapering off slowly—gradually reducing your coffee intake—may help reduce the discomfort of withdrawal. However, the unpleasant symptoms usually last for only a few days, and may be lessened in severity by doing such simple things as taking acetaminophen (avoid over-the-counter medication with added caffeine) and sipping a strong cup of peppermint tea.

If you're trying to avoid caffeine, keep in mind that it is added to many soft drinks, painkillers, diet pills, and over-the-counter stimulants. Try to buy only caffeine-free products.

Exercising first thing in the morning helps produce the endorphins that can relieve pain and give you a feeling of well-being.

*Help! During the winter, my skin gets dry and itchy.
Sometimes I even develop a form of eczema which is
very uncomfortable. What can I do?*

Cold weather and indoor heating, which zaps moisture
from the air, can cause skin to dry out. In the winter, many
people, like yourself, develop eczema, a mild rash characterized by rough, dry, scaly areas on the skin. External lubri-
cants (such as Curél, Alpha Keri, and Lubriderm) can help
reduce irritation and restore much needed moisture to the
skin. In addition, flaxseed oil capsules (1 capsule 3 times
daily) or 1 to 2 tablespoons of the liquid may also help to
keep you from drying out.

Don't forget to get enough beta-carotene, from either
food or a supplement, to help keep your skin healthy.

*I've tried to eat my daily quota of fiber, I really have!
But when I begin to load up on bran and beans, I
develop a bad case of stomach cramps and diarrhea.
Is my body trying to tell me to forget the fiber?*

Actually, I think your body is trying to tell you to take it
slow and easy. When many people hear that they are supposed to be eating around 30 grams of fiber daily, their initial reaction is to rush out and gobble up as much of the
stuff as is humanly possible. But that can be a big mistake. A
large quantity of fiber suddenly dumped down your gastrointestinal tract can be quite irritating. In fact, many fiber
neophytes complain of gas and bloating as well as general
gastric discomfort. To prevent having any problems, slowly
introduce fiber into your body until you gradually work
your way up to your optimum level. For example, begin by
eating a moderately high-fiber cereal, such as shredded

wheat or grape nuts (roughly 4 grams of fiber per serving) before trying a very high-fiber cereal, such as All-Bran with Extra Fiber (14 grams). If you're not used to eating salads, don't pile your plate sky high with goodies from the salad bar. Begin by eating one medium-size bowl of lettuce (with mixed, raw vegetables) before graduating to a dinner-size portion. The same is true for fruit—if you've rarely eaten cantaloupe before, don't start by eating a whole melon at a time. A quarter of a melon is enough to start.

Beans are a wonderful source of fiber and protein, but many people have difficulty digesting them because our bodies actually lack the enzyme to digest bean sugar. Soaking dried beans overnight and cooking them until they are well done will dispel most of the gas-producing sugar. In addition, add beans slowly to your diet, starting with ½ cup of cooked beans one or two times per week until your body adjusts to this new food. There is a product on the market that can aid in bean digestion—it works by providing an enzyme that helps the body break down the bean sugar. Many people swear by this product; however, it is made from a mold and could produce an allergic reaction in mold-sensitive individuals.

Since my son has started kindergarten, we're both constantly battling colds and sore throats. What's a mother to do?

It's normal for a kindergarten child to pick up a lot of colds; for the first time, he is being exposed to a lot of different viral and bacterial infections from the other children. Usually, by first or second grade, children get sick less often. It's also not unusual for colds to run their course through a family; however, it sounds as if your family is getting more than its fair share. Here are some things that you should do to keep infections at bay.

You and your son should increase your intake of vitamin C, nature's own immune booster. Eat lots of fruits and vegetables—strawberries, citrus fruits, cantaloupe, broccoli, and sweet red pepper are good choices. An added bonus: these foods are also rich in beta-carotene, which is also essential for a strong immune system.

Vitamin B_6 (found in fortified instant oatmeal and ready-to-eat cereals, liver, and chicken) is also important for proper immune function. Don't forget to get enough vitamin E—it can help the body produce more T cells, which ward off infection. Good sources of E include peanut butter, almonds, brown rice, oatmeal, and walnuts.

Everyone in your family should eat at least one 8-ounce container of low-fat or nonfat yogurt with live cultures daily (unless the family member is allergic to milk products). People who eat lots of yogurt have substantially higher levels of gamma-interferon, a substance produced by white blood cells, the body's own defense system, than those who don't eat yogurt.

Finally, if you are getting sick more often than normal, perhaps you should have your doctor check you for anemia. Excessive fatigue and lowered resistance to infection are signs that your body may be lacking iron, folic acid, copper, or B_{12}. A deficiency in any of these could result in a reduced number of red blood cells, which could throw your immune system out of whack.

I've noticed that my 12-year-old daughter is beginning to put on a few pounds. Frankly, I feel a bit guilty about it because my husband and I are both a bit

heavy and are not at all careful about what we eat.
I don't want my daughter to have a weight problem.
What can I do to help her without making her crazy?

Good question! About 15 percent of all adolescents—more girls than boys—are obese, that is, 15 to 20 percent above their normal body weight. The sedentary life-style of many adolescents (whose main activity is holding a telephone in one hand and a Nintendo control in the other), and the high-fat content of popular junk foods, such as candy bars and chips, are major culprits in adolescent obesity. Unfortunately, obese adolescents grow into obese adults. Now's the time to get your daughter back on track, and while you're doing it, you and your husband might as well go along for the ride.

In a way, you're lucky that you and your husband are overweight because you can shift the focus away from your daughter and on yourselves, which will make her feel less self-conscious. Explain to your daughter that you and your husband are worried about your health and therefore are putting yourselves on a healthy eating plan. (Don't use the "D" word, please.) Ask her to cooperate with you. Clean your pantry and refrigerator of high-fat junk food; replace it with low-fat snacks such as pretzels, air-popped popcorn, fresh fruit, frozen juice bars, no-fat frozen yogurt, and other satisfying but not fattening treats. Plan your menus carefully. Pasta with a low-fat tomato sauce, stir-fried beef with vegetables, and broiled chicken without skin are good main courses, but watch portion size. Learn to cook with legumes and grains—they're high in fiber, which will fill you up, but low in calories. Avoid fat-laden foods like hot dogs, french fries fried in oil (oven-baked fries are fine), and high-fat entrées like eggplant parmigiana that are soaked in oil and slathered with cheese. Replace sugary colas with flavored seltzer water, or make a "spritzer" out of seltzer and a splash of juice. If you eat out, choose a Japanese or Chinese restaurant that serves tasty but low-fat seafood, vegetable, or noodle dishes. Finally, and perhaps most important, don't forget to turn off the TV and start exercising. Physical activity will help the calories melt away for you, your husband, and your daughter.

CHAPTER 10

Staying Healthy, Feeling Young

At the turn of the century, the average life expectancy for a U.S. citizen was 47; today it is 75. But merely extending life span is not enough—the quality of those years is every bit as important as the quantity. Frankly, I believe that we can do a lot more to ensure a better quality of life as we age.

Here's the bad news: As it stands now, one out of three Americans will get cancer at some point in their lifetime, and in the twenty-first century, that number is expected to rise to one out of two. Nearly 60 percent of all people over 65 have high blood pressure, and nearly one third have heart disease. Forty-five percent of the elderly are on prescription drugs for ailments ranging from arthritis to hypertension to glaucoma.

Now for the good news: Growing older need not be synonymous with illness. It can and should be a productive, fulfilling time of life, that is, if you choose the right lifestyle. There is mounting evidence that diet, nutrition, and exercise can make a tremendous difference in how we age. In order to understand the importance of diet, let me first review some of the theories of why we age.

I. Free-Radical Theory of Aging

Proponents of the "free-radical" theory believe that aging is actually caused by molecules with unstable electrical charges called free radicals (the same culprits that I earlier noted may be responsible for atherosclerosis and many forms of cancer). Free radicals are constantly being produced by the body or, in some cases, are produced in the environment. For example, air contains oxygen, O_2, but when sunlight hits polluted air, O_2 is transformed into O_3, or ozone. Unlike O_2, O_3 is very unstable, which means that it is looking to combine with another molecule. Free radicals are highly reactive; they bounce around inside body cells causing damage to cell membranes, proteins, and DNA. Free radicals can also attack collagen, the glue that binds cells together, resulting in an increasing amount of fibrous tissue and blood cells in cell walls. The collagen becomes less flexible and the body begins to show signs of aging, such as stiff joints and wrinkled skin.

To combat free radicals, our bodies are constantly producing antioxidants or utilizing the antioxidants we obtain from nutrients. As we age, however, we begin to produce less antioxidants on our own, and in many cases, our diets are not sufficient to provide the additional antioxidant boost that we may need. Antioxidants include beta-carotene, vitamins C and E, zinc, and selenium.

II. The Immune Theory of Aging

As its name implies, the immune theory of aging focuses on the role of the immune system in the aging process. As we get older, our immune system becomes less efficient, leaving the body more vulnerable to infection. Also, our immune system has more difficulty differentiating between our own cells and those of invading organisms. Thus, a malfunctioning immune system may begin to attack its own tissues and organs, actually causing the problems it's supposed to prevent. Certain forms of diabetes and arthritis are linked to this kind of autoimmune disorder. The right vitamins and minerals can help to keep the immune system well functioning throughout our lifetime.

III. The RNA/DNA Theory of Aging

The nucleic acids, RNA (ribonucleic acid) and DNA (deoxyribonucleic acid), are the cellular components that control heredity and, subsequently, the body's ability to keep producing its inherited pattern. Because of RNA and DNA, we are capable of producing new cells after we are born. However, as we age, our cells become less capable of replenishing themselves. For example, a healthy child produces millions and millions of new cells daily to facilitate growth. If the child is injured or gets sick, he or she mends quickly. An elderly person, however, produces new cells at a much slower rate. Sores and cuts take longer to heal. Illness exacts a more devastating toll. When the body can't produce enough new cells to replace the old ones, we begin to see signs of aging, such as wrinkled, less supple skin or dark "age spots" on the back of the hands.

In his book *Nucleic Acid Therapy in Aging and Degenerative Disease,* Dr. Benjamin S. Frank reported that deteriorating cells can be "rejuvenated" if supplied with nucleic acids. Dr. Frank reported that within two months of receiving nucleic acid therapy, his patients had more energy and better-looking skin.

As soon as I started eating a diet high in nucleic acids many years ago, I noticed a dramatic difference in how I look and feel. I have heard similar stories from friends and clients. Good food sources of nucleic acids include sardines (particularly water-packed Portuguese sardines), seafood, mushrooms, green leafy vegetables, anchovies, and certain types of nutritional yeast which clearly say on the label "rich in RNA and DNA." (Gout and certain forms of arthritis may be aggravated by a diet rich in nucleic acids. If you have these conditions, check with your physician before eating these foods.)

Eating Less, Eating Better

Aging may also be caused by eating too much of the wrong things and too little of the right things. For example, people in Japan and Iceland on average outlive Americans by up to five years. I believe that diet is a major factor. People in these countries are heavy fish eaters, which means that their diets are low in saturated fat and high in omega-3 fatty acids. In addition, they eat less processed foods than people in the United States and consume more grains and vegetables.

Americans are consuming far too many calories, particularly in the form of empty calories, or calories low in nutrients. I have seen people literally gorge on 3000 to 4000 calories a day, and still not meet their basic RDA for many vitamins and minerals! Sugary sodas, snack foods, processed and fast foods can pack a caloric wallop without making a dent in terms of nutrition.

There is also some evidence that too many calories may hamper longevity. In a recent study at the Human Nutrition Research Center on Aging at Tufts University, one group of mice was fed a very nutritious but low-calorie diet, and another group as much food as they wanted. The mice on the low-calorie but healthy diet seemed to show less signs of wear and tear than the other mice, and actually lived 15 to 50 percent longer!

Are You Getting Enough of What You Need?

Despite our excesses, many older people are not getting enough of the nutrients they need. Studies show that many people over 60 are deficient in one or more essential vitamins and/or minerals. These shortages can seriously impair their mental or physical functioning.

The following are some of the major reasons that older people are at risk of not getting enough nutrients:

Inefficient Digestion

As we age, our digestive system gets less efficient. Thus even if we continue to eat a well-rounded diet, we may not have the ability to absorb the nutrients that we are taking in. For instance, many people over 50 may develop indigestion, characterized by gas and bloating after eating. If you have these symptoms, check with your physician—it could be a sign of an underlying medical problem. However, very often the indigestion is due to the inability of the body to produce enough hydrochloric acid (HCl) to break down food. A simple solution is to take an enzyme such as bromelin (derived from pineapple) or papain (derived from papaya) ½ hour either before or after eating. These natural enzymes will help the body break down food and utilize vitamins and minerals.

In general, to avoid indigestion, older people should not eat too much fat and protein, which are more difficult to digest than complex carbohydrates. In addition, eat slowly and avoid drinking very hot or very cold fluids, which can aggravate a strained stomach.

Poor Diet

Many older people, especially those who live alone, have very poor eating habits. As a result of illness or isolation, many older Americans don't bother cooking for themselves, but rely on convenience or processed foods, which are often lower in nutrients and higher in sugar and sodium. In addition, many older people skip meals altogether and, as a result, are poorly nourished.

Older patients in hospitals and nursing homes are not any better off. Institutional cooking is often bland and tasteless, which is another reason a patient or nursing home resident may not be eating all that he or she should.

Loss of Taste and Smell

Our senses of taste and smell decline with age. By around age 60, many older adults complain that food tastes bland and uninteresting. If you have this problem, try waking up your taste buds with a variety of new herbs and spices. A zinc supplement of zinc gluconate (15 to 60 mg) may also help.

Dental Pain

Gum disease, poorly fitted dentures, or other teeth or mouth problems could interfere with the ability to eat and enjoy food. Maintaining good dental health is essential; also a diet rich in flavonoids (found in fruits, especially citrus, and vegetables) can help strengthen gums.

Medications and Their Side Effects

Nearly half of all older Americans are on prescription medications (and countless millions on self-prescribed over-the-counter drugs). Some medications may actually cause an off taste in the mouth, which can impair the ability to discern different flavors. Even a routinely used drug such as aspirin can interfere with the ability to taste bitter flavors. If you are taking a drug that is interfering with your ability to enjoy food, talk to your physician. Certain medications can also interfere with the ability to absorb vitamins and nutrients. For example:

- Diuretics, or water pills, which are given to control high blood pressure, can sap the body of potassium, B-complex, magnesium, and zinc.
- People who routinely take laxatives—which is not uncommon among older people—can also suffer from a loss of potassium.
- The cancer drug methotrexate (which is also used for psoriasis) can destroy folic acid.
- Aspirin can increase the excretion of vitamin C from the body.
- Cortisone and prednisone, often used for arthritis pain, can lower zinc levels.

◆ Cholestyramine, given to lower cholesterol, can rob the body of vitamins A, D, E, and K and potassium.

And finally, the most commonly used drug of all, alcohol, which is present in many over-the-counter cold medications, can reduce blood levels of vitamins A, B_1, B_2, biotin, choline, niacin, vitamin B_{15} (pangamic acid, an antioxidant), folic acid, magnesium, and vitamin C.

Older people are not just getting too much alcohol through their cold medicines, many are alcohol abusers. Due to isolation and loneliness, millions of older Americans are problem drinkers. To compound the problem, as we age, our bodies produce less of the enzyme required to break down alcohol. As a result, we feel the effects of alcohol much faster. Alcohol not only robs our bodies of vital nutrients, but can severely hamper our ability to think clearly and perform tasks such as driving. Therefore, older people in particular should be extremely careful about alcohol intake.

50-Plus Checklist

After age 50, people need to make sure that they are getting the nutrition they need to stay vital and healthy. Here are some of the vitamins, minerals, and nutrients you need now more than ever.

Beta-carotene

Few Americans get the full 10,000 IU (6 mg) of beta-carotene (nearly twice the RDA) that many experts say are needed to protect against cancer and heart disease. It is especially important that people over 50, who are at greater risk of these diseases, eat enough beta-carotene-rich foods, such as dark green leafy vegetables and yellow and orange fruits and vegetables.

Thiamine (B₁)

Low levels of this vitamin can cause subtle changes in brain function among older people which can affect their ability to think clearly and perform tasks well. A good B-complex vitamin will provide ample amounts of B_1.

Vitamin B₆

B_6 increases immunity for older people. A recent study found that those with low levels of this vitamin had depressed immune systems. Be sure to get 50 mg of B_6 daily.

Riboflavin (B₂)

Active older women in particular need more of this vitamin, which is important for stamina. I recommend taking 50 mg daily.

Vitamin B₁₂

Older people have difficulty absorbing B_{12}. As a result, many people over 60 suffer from B_{12} deficiency, which can result in confusion, mood changes, and other symptoms that could easily be mistaken for senility. A B_{12} supplement can reverse these symptoms. I recommend the nasal gel or the sublingual form, which bypasses the stomach and is absorbed directly into the bloodstream. Take 400 mcg nasal gel every 2 to 3 days, or 1000 to 2000 mcg of the sublingual form daily.

Folic Acid

Older people in particular do not get enough of this B vitamin, which helps to prevent anemia, certain forms of cancer and may even protect against heart disease. Good sources include green leafy vegetables, wheat germ, asparagus, and chicken liver. If you use a supplement, take 400 mcg daily.

Vitamin C

You need more of this antioxidant, which can help protect against cancer, heart disease, and even the common cold. Eat lots of food rich in C or take a supplement. I recommend taking 1000 to 2000 mg daily. Esterified, timed-release vitamin C is gentler on the stomach.

Vitamin D

Recent studies show that older people get only half the vitamin D they should. Women in particular, who are at risk of osteoporosis, need to take this vitamin, which can help in calcium absorption. In addition, people who are housebound and don't get enough sunshine, which stimulates the body to produce vitamin D, may also be short of this vitamin. Food sources of vitamin D include fortified milk and fatty fish. I recommend taking a supplement of 400 IU daily.

Vitamin E (Tocopherol)

To improve circulation, reduce your risk of heart attack, and beef up your immune system, I recommend that everyone over 50 take a supplement of 400 IU D-alpha Tocopherol, the most effective form of Vitamin E. The dried form is better absorbed.

Calcium

Women who are not on estrogen replacement therapy need to take at least 1500 mg of this mineral daily. Your best bet is to take a supplement of 1000 to 1200 mg in addition to eating more nonfat or low-fat dairy products.

Fiber

An adequate amount of fiber can improve bowel function (so you won't need laxatives), reduce blood pressure, and protect against cancer and heart disease. All it takes is about 30 grams of fiber daily, which is easy to obtain if you eat a diet rich in grains, fruits, and vegetables.

Selenium

This mineral is an antioxidant that protects against various cancers. Many Americans do not get enough selenium in their diets. Selenium can be found in garlic, onions, and broccoli, as well as other food. I recommend that people over 50 take 100 mcg daily. (Doses over 5 mg can be toxic.)

What You Don't Know
Can Hurt You
■ ■ ■

CHAPTER 11

What Jack Sprat (and His Wife) Didn't Know About Fats

Fat and cholesterol are two of the most confusing subjects for health-conscious consumers, and no wonder. One week you hear that margarine is good for your heart, and the next week you hear that margarine is bad. For years, you've been warned to steer clear of nuts because of their high-fat content, and the latest studies now show that nuts can cut cholesterol. To add to your bewilderment, your physician recently told you that even though your total cholesterol was low, your level of good cholesterol (HDL) was too low, and he wants you to try to raise it!

If you're perplexed by all of these things, you're not alone. I am frequently asked questions about fat and cholesterol, and in this chapter, I will try to answer these questions as simply as possible.

What's so bad about fat?

First, I want to stress that fat is not the enemy. In fact, fat is an important part of the human body. A woman's body is composed of about 25 to 35 percent fatty tissue; a man's body has about 10 percent less. Body fat has several important jobs. It carries fat-soluble vitamins (A, D, E, and K) throughout the body and provides a reserve of energy in times of famine. It also protects and insulates body organs and is essential for the production of sex hormones.

Fat becomes a problem only when there's too much of it. A diet high in fat has been linked to an increased risk of various forms of cancer, including colon and rectal cancer, prostate cancer, and recurrence of breast cancer. A high-fat diet has also been associated with an increased risk of heart attack and stroke. The average American diet is very high in fat: Americans consume nearly 40 percent of their daily calories in the form of fat. The U.S. Surgeon General and the National Academy of Sciences Committee on Diet and Health recommend that you consume no more than 30 percent of your calories in fat. Other experts—the late Nathan Pritikin and Dean Ornish, M.D.—feel that even 30 percent is too high, and recommend as little as 10 or 15 percent of fat in the total diet. I, myself, would be happy if people could keep their daily fat intake down to around 20 percent of their total calories.

What is cholesterol and what does it have to do with fat?

Cholesterol is a waxy, yellowish, fatlike substance that is produced primarily in the liver and in lesser quantities in the intestines and specialized cells throughout the body. Like fat, cholesterol is an important part of the body. It is essential for the production of sex hormones, it is required for the synthesis of vitamin D, and it is needed to produce cell membranes and the myelin sheath, the fatty coat that surrounds nerves.

In addition to being produced by the body, cholesterol is also found in certain foods. For example, the average egg contains about 213 mg of cholesterol; a 3-ounce hamburger contains 76 mg. However, you don't have to eat extra cholesterol to meet the body's needs; even if you had a cholesterol-free diet, the body would produce enough to function quite nicely. Certain types of fats found in food can also trigger the production of cholesterol within the body.

Similar to fat, cholesterol causes problems only when there is too much of it. An excess of blood cholesterol can promote the formation of plaque, a substance that clogs arteries and prevents the normal flow of blood throughout the body. If the artery leading to the heart becomes clogged with plaque, it can result in a heart attack.

The American Heart Association recommends that you eat no more than 300 mg of cholesterol each day.

How do we know that high cholesterol causes heart disease?

Several major studies confirm the link between heart disease and cholesterol. A major study of nineteen countries, sponsored by the World Health Organization, showed that countries that consumed the highest amount of saturated fat had the highest blood cholesterol levels (typically, over 250 mg/dl) and the highest rate of heart disease. Another study, in Japan/Honolulu/San Francisco, examined the eating habits of three groups of Japanese men. The first group lived in Japan and ate the traditional Japanese diet, which is low in fat; the second group were native Japanese who had migrated to Hawaii and were presumably eating what the Hawaiians eat; and the third group were native Japanese who had moved to San Francisco and were eating the typical high-fat American diet. After ten years, the Japanese men living in Japan had the lowest levels of cholesterol and the lowest incidence of heart disease. Those in Hawaii had somewhat higher rates of cholesterol and heart disease, but those living in San Francisco had the highest rates of both. Studies like this show a direct connection between diet, cholesterol, and heart disease.

What is the difference between "good" and "bad" cholesterol?

Within the body, cholesterol needs to be metabolized— that is, broken down into a form that can be used by the body and sent to the cells that need it. The excess is stored. The liver repackages cholesterol in the form of LDL ("bad cholesterol") or low-density lipoprotein. LDL delivers the cholesterol to the tissues for cell membrane production, repair, and production of sex hormones. Some of the LDL is reduced further to HDL ("good cholesterol") or high-density lipoprotein, which carries the excess cholesterol back to the intestine to be excreted from the body.

LDL, the body's major carrier of cholesterol, is believed to be a leading culprit in the formation of plaque deposits. As LDLs circulate throughout the blood, they latch onto special receptor sites in the cells that need them. When cells have enough cholesterol, they stop producing receptor sites, allowing the LDLs to remain in the blood. Researchers believe that a high level of LDLs in the blood can cause injury to the innermost layer of the artery wall, thus causing atherosclerosis or narrowing of the artery. A new theory suggests that LDLs may become oxidized by free radicals, which the cells within the lining wall interpret as injury, and thus, send for help in the form of white cells called monocytes. These cells stick to the cell lining, and attract other cells, which all contribute to the formation of plaque.

What is a healthy cholesterol level?

An overall cholesterol under 200 mg/dl is considered to be the ideal number and 200–239 is considered to be borderline high. Anything above that is bona fide high. However, an elevated overall cholesterol (up to about 240) may still be considered good as long as the levels of HDL are proportionally high:

- The ratio between total cholesterol and HDL should not exceed 6 : 1. Therefore, if a man has a total cholesterol level of 240, but an HDL of 60, the ratio is 4 : 1, which is quite good.
- The ratio between LDL and HDL ideally should be 3 : 1, but should not exceed 4 : 1. For example, if the LDL is 120, the HDL should be 40 or better.

According to the American Heart Association, even a low cholesterol level can signal danger if the HDL is too low. In fact, recent findings show that levels of HDL under 35 appear to increase the risk of having a heart attack. Regular exercise, diet, and supplementary niacin can raise HDL.

What are triglycerides?

Triglycerides are a type of fat that can be found in the blood and are measured by a special test. Studies show that triglyceride levels of more than 190 mg/dl for women and 400 mg/dl for men increase the odds of developing heart disease.

What are the benefits of lowering a high cholesterol?

The Coronary Prevention Trial of 1984 provides the answer to your question. In this study, 3800 men with elevated cholesterol levels were given either a cholesterol-lowering drug or a placebo. The men who took the drug experienced a 9 percent drop in cholesterol and reduced their risk of heart attack by 19 percent as compared with the group not on the cholesterol-lowering drug. Based on this study, for every 1 percent decline in cholesterol, you gain a 2 percent decrease in your risk of having a heart attack. (I'm not suggesting that people should take cholesterol-lowering drugs; in fact, in many cases, many foods and vitamins work just as well and have far fewer side effects.)

Good Fats, Bad Fats— A Guide to Dietary Fats

Not all fats are equal. There are many different types of fat in the food we eat; some fats are actually good for us, and some are downright dangerous. The following section outlines the different types of fat—the good, the bad, and the terrible.

Dietary fat comes in three varieties: saturated fats, polyunsaturated fats, and monounsaturated fats. These three fats differ in chemical structure, notably in the number of hydrogen molecules. The more hydrogen molecules, the more saturated the fat. Therefore, polyunsaturated or monounsaturated fats have fewer hydrogen molecules.

Fat is very fattening: a fat gram is equal to 9 calories, regardless of the type of fat. (Protein and carbohydrate have 4 calories per gram.)

Saturated Fats

Saturated fats are found primarily in food of animal origin, such as fatty cuts of beef, lard, whole milk dairy products, and lamb. There is less saturated fat in chicken, fish, and lean cuts of beef. Plant sources of saturated fat include peanut butter and coconut. Saturated fat tends to be solid at room temperature. The problem with saturated fat is that it stimulates the body to increase its production of cholesterol, especially the bad or LDL cholesterol.

PERSONAL ADVICE Try to limit your daily intake of saturated fat to under 10 percent of your total calories. Eat only the leanest cuts of beef and skinless white meat poultry. Cook fish in an oil-free environment. Watch your portion size! (A healthy-size portion is roughly the size of a deck of cards.)

Polyunsaturated Fats

Polyunsaturated fats are found in vegetable oils and margarine made from plant sources. These fats are the body's main source of linoleic acid, which is necessary for the formation of cells and the normal functioning of the nervous system.

Highly polyunsaturated oils, such as safflower, corn, and sunflower oil, have been shown to reduce blood cholesterol levels. However, certain types of polyunsaturated oils can actually raise cholesterol. Some polyunsaturated oils and all margarines undergo a process called hydrogenation to make them useful for baking and to increase their shelf life. This process creates substances called *trans*-fatty acids which act like saturated fats in the body in that they stimulate the production of cholesterol. Studies show that people who eat a lot of hydrogenated polyunsaturated oil and margarine have higher cholesterol levels than those who don't. (No, this doesn't mean that you can switch back to butter; butter is just as bad, if not worse.)

In addition, a diet high in polyunsaturated oil has been linked to certain forms of cancer and the formation of gall-stones. Several studies have shown that polyunsaturated oil is prone to oxidative damage, a process in the body that may be responsible for some forms of heart disease and cancer.

PERSONAL ADVICE Stick to unhydrogenated oils. Buy only unhydrogenated, liquid margarine in a squeeze bottle and use it sparingly. Diet margarine and liquid margarine in squeeze bottles have less *trans*-fatty acids. Try not to consume more than 10 percent of your calories in the form of polyunsaturated fat.

Monounsaturated Fats

Monounsaturated fats are found in common cooking oils, including olive oil, canola oil, peanut oil, and some forms of sunflower and safflower oil. Monounsaturated oil—olive oil in particular—has a beneficial effect on blood cholesterol. Several studies have shown that although olive oil has no effect on total cholesterol, it can increase the amount of HDL or good cholesterol. In addition, researchers in Israel recently discovered that olive oil was prone to less oxidative damage than polyunsaturated oil; oxidative damage of blood lipids is believed to be a major risk factor for developing atherosclerosis.

Good sources of monounsaturated oil also include almonds, avocado, cashews, and peanuts.

PERSONAL ADVICE Try to replace the other fats in your diet with more monounsaturated fats, especially olive oil. As good as olive oil is, it is still high in calories and should not be used with a heavy hand. One or two tablespoons a day in cooking or on your salad is quite enough.

CAUTION

READ THE LABELS Commercially prepared and processed foods may be very high in fats of all kinds, but especially in saturated fat and hydrogenated polyunsaturated fat. In particular, avoid croissants, doughnuts, muffins, butter rolls, and biscuits from bakeries—they are very high in fat. Look for packaged products that are low in fat, and use canola, safflower, or only partially hydrogenated oils. Tropical oils (such as palm and coconut oil) can, similarly to saturated fat, raise cholesterol.

Fast Food: Worse Than Margarine

The worst offender of all may be the hydrogenated vegetable oils that are used for frying in fast-food restaurants. These oils contain higher levels of *trans*-fatty acids than margarine. Don't eat them!

A Fishy Tale: The Omega-3s

Omega-3 fatty acids are a form of polyunsaturated fat and have received a great deal of publicity lately because of their beneficial effect on the body. These fatty acids are found primarily in fatty fish and flaxseed oil.

Scientists speculate that, early in human development, our original diet included many more foods rich in omega-3s. Today, many of us are not getting enough of this important fatty acid. Omega-3s have been shown to do the following:

Coronary Artery Disease

Numerous studies show that fish oil lowers total cholesterol and LDL cholesterol among people with slightly high cholesterol who substitute fatty fish for saturated fat in their diet. (Substitute is the operative word here—if you add fatty fish but do not decrease saturated fat, you will experience a slight increase in cholesterol.) Omega-3 fatty acid also lowers triglycerides in patients with elevated triglycerides, which is a particular risk factor for women for developing heart disease.

Recent studies show that omega-3 fatty acid inhibits the production of platelet-derived growth factor, a substance believed to be responsible for formation of plaque deposits in arteries.

Omega-3 fatty acid also lowers blood levels of fibrinogen and thromboxane. Fibrinogen is a substance produced in the body that is necessary for the proper clotting of blood. High levels are associated with the formation of blood clots, which can lead to stroke and higher rates of atherosclerosis. Thromboxane causes blood vessels to constrict, which can cause high blood pressure.

Anti-inflammatory Effect

Omega-3 fatty acids have anti-inflammatory properties, that is, they inhibit the biochemical pathway in the cells that triggers an inflammatory reaction. Omega-3s have been used successfully to treat symptoms associated with arthritis, lupus, psoriasis, ulcerative colitis, and other inflammatory diseases.

Cancer Protector

Although some polyunsaturated fats stimulate tumor growth, several studies show that fish oil inhibits the growth of cancerous tumors in animals.

Pregnancy

Omega-3 fatty acids have been used in high-risk pregnancies to prevent miscarriage; researchers believe that they may prevent the formation of blood clots in the placenta, and also help to keep blood pressure lower by reducing the levels of thromboxane.

PERSONAL ADVICE Eat 2 to 3 fish meals a week or take flaxseed or a fish oil supplement.

The New Fake Fats: Are They Safe?

More and more, foods with added synthetic fats are beginning to appear on supermarket shelves. Their appeal is obvious: Fat adds texture and flavor to food, but it also adds lots of calories. If a no-calorie or low-calorie synthetic fat could do the same thing, obviously it's worth cheering about. But I'm not cheering about all of these fake fats. Fake fats are made from a wide variety of ingredients, ranging from egg whites to modified food starch, which are fairly benign, to some that I consider to be potentially problematic. For example, gum arabic and carrageenan, which are frequently used to add a creamy texture to low-fat foods, can cause allergic symptoms and other adverse reactions in some people. Also, although these additives require FDA approval, I'm not sure that all of them have been adequately tested. For example, in 1987, Procter and Gamble petitioned the FDA to approve a new product called Olestra. The Center for Science in the Public Interest requested that the FDA not grant approval because of the lack of testing on Olestra. According to CSPI, preliminary testing showed that Olestra might increase the risk of cancer and birth defects among humans. The FDA has held up approval on Olestra, but I'm concerned that other substitutes have slipped through. Keep in mind that we really have no way of knowing the long-term effects of such a relatively new product.

I think your best bet is to steer clear of these phony fats, and use natural substitutions in your own cooking and baking. For example, adding a cup of oatmeal to meatloaf is a natural and healthy way to reduce fat. Cooking with applesauce or plain yogurt can often reduce fat in a recipe without compromising moisture or flavor. Make your own frozen yogurt or ice milk using no-fat yogurt or low-fat milk. There are lots of ways that you can satisfy your fat craving without succumbing to these new chemical concoctions.

A Word About Nuts

Nuts are a food that breaks all of the rules. Nuts derive between 70 and 90 percent of their calories from fat, which means that they're bad for you, right? Wrong. It appears that the polyunsaturated fat in nuts has a beneficial effect on cholesterol. A recent study showed that people who went on a high-walnut diet (that is, 20 percent of their daily calories came from walnuts) experienced a 12 percent decline in total cholesterol. We know from another major study of more than 26,000 members of the Seventh-Day Adventist Church that those people who ate peanuts, walnuts, or almonds at least five times a week had an average life span of seven years longer than the general population, and a substantially lower rate of heart attack. Keep in mind that eating nuts may not be the only reason why these folks fared so well. Seventh-Day Adventists don't drink, smoke, or eat meat, which may all contribute to a healthier than normal life-style. However, researchers still believe that nuts play a strong role in their increased longevity.

If you want to add nuts to your diet, keep in mind that you must cut out an equal number of calories to compensate for the additional nuts, or you will gain weight very quickly. Just one ounce of walnuts is 170 calories—that's nothing to be taken lightly.

Common Food Fallacies

♦ Spicy food can cause ulcers.

For years, people have blamed ulcers on everything from stress to spice (as in hot chili, pepperoni pizza, Szechuan food, etc.). However, recent findings suggest that in at least 90 percent of all cases the real culprit is a bacterium called *Campylobacter pylori*, and the cure is a simple antibiotic. Although most people harbor these bacteria, only a small fraction will actually develop ulcers. In fact, although spicy food may aggravate the condition in a handful of people, genetics may play a more important role in determining who actually gets ulcers. Smoking, coffee (including decaffeinated), and alcohol can all contribute to an ulcer flare-up.

♦ Frozen yogurt isn't a "real" dessert; it's a health food.

Although most frozen yogurt is lower in fat and calories than many brands of ice cream, it is loaded with sugar. Furthermore, it does not contain the same level of active cultures as plain yogurt, and does not offer the same health benefits. Don't gorge on frozen yogurt in the mistaken belief that you are eating a "health food," stick to a ½ cup serving of the solid variety, or one dish of the soft variety. Also, watch out for the toppings—granola, M & M's, and chocolate sprinkles, which are frequently offered at yogurt shops—they can add both fat and calories.

♦ Juice is better than eating fruits or vegetables.

"Juicing" has become quite a fad in recent years as more and more people invest in juicers. Although drinking juice is certainly better than drinking soft drinks, keep in mind that juice can add on a lot of extra calories in the course of the day. For example, a cup of apple juice is 115 calories and a cup of orange juice is 110. Unlike eating fresh fruits or vegetables, juice does not contain fiber, nor can it give you that feeling of fullness which can help prevent excess eating.

♦ Sandwiches are fattening; salads are not.

Sometimes yes, sometimes no. A plain salad with cut-up fresh vegetables topped off with a lemon, olive oil, or a touch of low-fat dressing is a sensible, low-calorie food option. And it's certainly better than a pastrami sandwich. However, many people mistakenly believe that the salad they concoct at their local salad bar—a handful of lettuce leaves smothered with bits of cheese, buttery croutons, crumbled bacon, blue cheese dressing, and mayonnaise-laden tuna salad—is actually a good option. It's not. A better choice would be a few slices of white meat turkey on whole grain bread, with mustard, lettuce, and tomato.

♦ Anything "natural" is healthy.

Natural is not synonymous with healthy. In fact, many potent carcinogens are present in "natural" foods. For example, aflatoxin, a mold commonly found on peanuts, in peanut butter, and on other fruits and vegetables, is a known carcinogen. Cooked meat contains carcinogenic compounds. In most cases, our bodies are able to destroy these carcinogens before they do their harm; however, good nutrition can boost our defenses against these troublemakers.

CHAPTER 12

Food Additives

There are hundreds of products that are added to food, and most of us—unless we are avid readers of the fine print—are totally unaware of them. Food additives may be used to retard spoilage, enhance flavor, increase shelf life, or even as a "filler" to help a manufacturer cut costs. During the course of the day, it is possible to consume scores of chemicals. Although most are regarded as safe—and, indeed, many are harmless—some are not so benign. Here is a list of the twenty food additives that I feel should be avoided or that can cause problems for many people. Nearly all of these additives are on the FDA's GRAS (Generally Recognized as Safe) list, which means that they are allowed to be sold without FDA approval and are consumed in unlimited quantity. Of course, a product can lose its GRAS rating if it's proven to be unsafe; however, millions of people may still be exposed to it before it is restricted or taken off the market.

Earl's "Terrible Twenty"

1. Acacia Gum (Gum Arabic)

This additive, which is often used in cake frostings, gum, and soft drinks, can cause mild to severe asthma attacks and rashes in humans. This additive has caused fatalities in pregnant animals.

I feel that acacia gum should be avoided by allergic individuals and by pregnant women, since it might possibly cause birth defects in susceptible individuals. Nursing mothers and women who are trying to conceive should probably steer clear of this one too.

2. Alginic Acid

This additive is found in ice cream, cheese spreads, salad dressings, and the like. Preliminary studies show that alginic acid may cause abnormal fetal development, and therefore I believe it should be avoided by women who are trying to conceive, and by already pregnant or nursing mothers.

3. Aluminum

Aluminum is widely used in many products, from white flour (to prevent caking) to processed cheeses (to facilitate melting) and toothpaste (as an abrasive). Although this theory is controversial, many experts believe that aluminum is associated with senile dementia and memory problems and, in fact, may be a cause of Alzheimer's disease. In addition, aluminum may cause kidney problems, mouth ulcers, gastrointestinal problems such as colitis, and may interfere with the normal absorption of other minerals. Until further testing is done to certify the safety of aluminum, I would avoid it.

4. Artificial Color

Artificial color additives are widely used in the food supply—so widely used in fact, that it's very hard to avoid them altogether. However, I still try to limit my intake and I advise others to do the same. Children are especially susceptible to additives, which may contribute to hyperactivity and learning disorders. If your kids are constantly bouncing off the walls, check their diet for artificial color additives. Sticking to fresh, unprocessed foods, or foods that are additive-free, will reduce the amount of additives in the diet.

5. *Benzaldehyde*

This additive, which is used in many processed foods, can cause depression in some people.

6. *Benzoic Acid*

This common additive, which is found in many jellies, jams, margarine and soft drinks, among other foods, may cause skin rashes, gastrointestinal upset in people of all age groups, and hyperactivity in children. Avoid it if you can.

7. *BHA or BHT (Butylated Hydroxyanisole or Butylated Hydroxytoluene)*

This additive, which is banned in England, may cause liver and kidney damage, behavioral problems in children, and can weaken the immune system.

8. *Brominated Vegetable Oil*

This additive may cause birth defects and growth problems in children and is considered unsafe by the FDA. However, it is still used in some foods and, therefore, should be avoided by pregnant women, nursing mothers, and children.

9. Carrageenan

Carrageenan, which is used as a thickening agent, may cause ulcerative colitis and colitis, and is a suspected cancer-producing agent.

10. Confectioners' Glaze

Confectioners' glaze is widely used on candy and drugs to provide a shiny coating. No studies have been done to evaluate this additive's safety in food use. Therefore, I think it's advisable not to use it.

11. EDTA (Ethylenediaminetetraacetic Acid-Salts)

This commonly used preservative may cause skin irritations, kidney damage, gastrointestinal upset, and mineral imbalances.

12. Hydrolyzed Vegetable Protein

This additive has two strikes against it. First, it contains MSG and is high in salt. Second, it may cause brain and nervous system damage in infants.

13. Iron Salts (Ferric Pyrophosphate, Ferric Sodium Pyrophosphate, Ferrous Lactate)

Iron salts are added to enriched breads and cereals, and other grains. I have several problems with this additive. First, I don't believe that it has been adequately tested for safety. Second, recent studies show that too much iron can increase your risk of having a heart attack. It's one thing to take an iron supplement when you need one; it's another to have one shoved down your unsuspecting throat. In particular, I don't recommend this additive for pregnant women, people with ulcers, or people with a condition called hemochromatosis, for whom even a normal intake of iron can be toxic.

14. Monoglycerides and Diglycerides, Acetylated Monoglycerides and Diglycerides

This additive, which is found in soy, corn, peanut, or fat based products may cause allergic reactions in some people.

15. Monosodium Glutamate (MSG)

MSG gained notoriety when it became linked to "Chinese restaurant syndrome," a condition associated with heart palpitations, headaches, and muscular weakness that occurs following a meal containing this additive, a favorite of Chinese chefs. In addition, MSG may cause nausea, high blood pressure, itching and other allergic reactions. Anyone who has ever felt light-headed or sick after eating Chinese food should avoid this additive. I also think that pregnant or lactating women should steer clear of MSG.

16. Nitrates

These additives prevent botulism, which is why they are used in so many foods. However, they form the powerful cancer-causing agent nitrosamine in the stomach, and can be very dangerous. Therefore, avoid them or limit your intake.

17. Paraffins (Wax)

Waxes, classified as chemical preservatives, are widely used on fruits, vegetables, and candy to make them shiny and pretty and to retard moisture loss and spoilage. Waxes are made from vegetable oils, palm oil derivatives, synthetic resins (also used in car and floor wax), as well as other materials. Some people, notably those who are allergic to aspirin, may be sensitive to many waxes, depending on their ingredients. These people should peel their fruits and vegetables or buy organic produce. In addition, waxes can seal in insecticides and fungicides, making it impossible to wash them off. If possible, buy your produce from a local farm or farmer's market where the fruits and vegetables are sold quickly, and may not be that heavily waxed. If you can't shop at a farmer's market, or if the produce sold at the market is heavily waxed, talk to your local supermarket manager or greengrocer about carrying a line of organic produce.

18. Potassium Bromate

Frequently used in baked products, this additive can cause nervous system or kidney disorders and gastrointestinal upset. It may also be carcinogenic. Try to avoid it.

19. Propyl Gallate

This additive has been associated with kidney and liver problems and gastrointestinal disturbances. I don't feel that propyl gallate has been properly tested, and that's why I think it should be avoided if possible. It is also usually found in combination with BHT or BHA, which may compound the potential problems caused by these additives.

(Propyl gallate has been banned in England from baby food or foods marketed to children.)

20. Sulfites

These additives lost their GRAS rating because they can cause a severe allergic reaction in asthmatics or highly allergic people. In fact, several deaths have been attributed to sulfites. Sulfites are used at salad bars to prevent discoloration of vegetables, in many wines, and as preservatives in many different foods. If a salad bar or greengrocer uses sulfites, by law they most post a sign warning consumers. However, the produce may have been treated before it even arrives at the greengrocery; therefore, people who are sensitive to sulfites should never graze at a salad bar. Sulfites also deplete food of vitamin B_1.

People who are sulfite-sensitive should carry a sulfite test strip, which they can purchase at their local pharmacy. The strip will turn bright red when touched by sulfite-containing food.

CHAPTER 13

Reading Between the Lines: Understanding Labels

In January 1992, the USDA issued its final rule on "Nutrition Labeling of Meat and Poultry Products," which took effect in 1994. Most meat and poultry products, except for raw, single-ingredient products, must include nutrition labels—packages of chili and hot dogs, for example, must bear nutrition labeling panels. (Products produced by small businesses or sold in small packages of under ½ ounce may be exempt.)

By 1994, all processed foods regulated by the Food and Drug Administration were required to post new and more detailed nutrition labels on their packages. (Previously, nutrition labels were purely voluntary, and in fact, one in five items sold did not provide a label.) These labels are a mixed blessing: based on the theory that overconsumption, not underconsumption, is the basic problem with the American diet, they exclude information that was once included on many packages, such as the level of B vitamins (unless a food is fortified or a manufacturer claims that a food is a good source of vitamin B). On the positive side, the labels include a great deal more information on fat, cholesterol, and fiber (most Americans are woefully low on fiber). However, this information is useful only if you understand how to use it.

Accompanying is a sample of one of the labels you're likely to see and how to decode it.

Nutrition Facts

Serving Size 1 cup (253g)
Servings Per Container 4

Amount Per Serving

Calories 260	Calories from Fat 70

	% Daily Value*
Total Fat 8g	**13%**
Saturated Fat 3g	**17%**
Cholesterol 130mg	**44%**
Sodium 1010mg	**42%**
Total Carbohydrate 22g	**7%**
Dietary Fiber 9g	**36%**
Sugars 4g	
Protein 25g	

Vitamin A	35%	•	Vitamin C	2%
Calcium	6%	•	Iron	30%

*Percent Daily Values are based on a 2,000 calorie diet. Your daily values may be higher or lower depending on your calorie needs:

	Calories:	2,000	2,500
Total Fat	Less than	65g	80g
Sat Fat	Less than	20g	25g
Cholesterol	Less than	300mg	300mg
Sodium	Less than	2,400mg	2,400mg
Total Carbohydrate		300g	375g
Dietary Fiber		25g	30g

Calories per gram:
Fat 9 • Carbohydrate 4 • Protein 4

Sample Label
(Consult FDA regulation for specific requirements on type size, spacing and other graphic elements.)

Where's the Beef?
Reading the Labels

Serving Size: No more sleight of hand. In the past, manufacturers could make a food appear to be lower in calories or fat by cutting the serving size. Serving sizes are now standardized, based on surveys that show the amount of a particular food that a person actually eats. In addition, the statistics on the food must reflect the amount of food in the serving size. For example, if a slice of cheese is ¾ ounce, the statistics on the label cannot reflect a 1-ounce serving.

Calories: The labels must divulge the caloric content of food, as well as how many calories come from fat of all kinds.

% Daily Value: The labels must reflect how a particular food affects an individual's daily food intake. The standard is based on a 2000-calorie diet. Therefore, if you're eating 2000 calories a day, according to the food guidelines no more than 30 percent, or under 700 calories a day, should be in the form of fat of any kind. (1 fat gram = 9 calories.) In this case, 8 grams is roughly 13 percent of your day's fat allocation. Although that may sound low, keep in mind, that this is just one food and fat calories add up rather quickly.

If you're eating less than 2000 calories a day, then 8 grams of fat will be somewhat more than 13 percent of your daily fat intake. If you're eating more, it will be somewhat less. (See chart on the bottom of the label.)

Total Fat: The labels not only include total fat but give the amount of saturated fat. No more than 10 percent of total daily calories should come from saturated fat. In this case, 3 grams of saturated fat equals 17 percent of the daily intake. Manufacturers can add polyunsaturated fats, mono-unsaturated fats, and *trans*-fatty acids.

Cholesterol: People are advised to eat no more than 300 mg of cholesterol daily. Therefore, 130 mg is nearly half of the daily allowance.

Sodium: People are advised to restrict sodium to 2400 mg a day. Under *% Daily Value,* you can see that 1010 mg is nearly half your daily allotment.

Total Carbohydrate: Roughly 60 percent of total calories should come from carbohydrate. In this meal, you have used up 7 percent of your daily total.

Dietary Fiber: Based on these numbers, people should eat 11.5 grams of fiber for every 1000 calories consumed. In this case, 9 grams provides more than a third of your needs.

Sugars: This measure is somewhat confusing because it includes naturally occurring sugars as well as added sugars. (There is no daily value for sugar.)

Protein: Some manufacturers may include protein, but they don't have to. The daily value for protein has been set at 50 grams for a 2000-calorie diet, which is less than what Americans eat.

Nutrients (Vitamins and Minerals): These figures are based on the USRDA.

What's in a Name?
Understanding the New Jargon

Prior to these federal regulations, manufacturers could declare any food "Lite" or "Lean" or "Low Fat." According to current rules, these and other similar terms are strictly defined.

Low fat: For a product to boast that it is low fat, it must contain 3 grams of fat or less per normal serving.

Lean: This term refers to meat or poultry with less than 10 grams of fat, less than 4 grams of saturated fat, and less than 95 mg of cholesterol per 100 grams. (A brand name containing lean, such as Lean Cuisine, can continue using its name even if it doesn't meet this criterion, if it was in use prior to November 27, 1991.)

Extra lean: To earn this label, meat or poultry must have less than 5 grams of fat, less than 2 grams of saturated fat, and less than 95 mg of cholesterol per 100 grams.

Low in calories: An individual food described as low calorie cannot contain more than 40 calories per normal serving.

Light (Lite): This term can be used for foods that have one-third fewer calories than a comparable product, or have half the fat content. (The label must specify which.) If the word *light* is used to describe taste, smell, or color, it must clearly state exactly what the term *light* is referring to. Light can also refer to foods that have half the sodium of a normal product, but it must clearly state: "Light in sodium."

Fat-free: This term may be used to describe a food that has 0.5 gram fat per serving (and no added oil or fat).

Reduced fat: Has no more than half the fat of an identified comparable food.

Low sodium: This means 140 mg or less per average serving.

Low cholesterol: This means that a food contains no more than 20 mg of cholesterol per typical serving.

Cholesterol-free: This term describes any food that has 2 mg or less of cholesterol per serving, and less than 2 grams of saturated fat per serving. (Saturated fat stimulates the production of cholesterol in the body.)

"Good" source: A food can be called a good source of a vitamin or nutrient if it provides at least 10 percent of the daily value.

"High" source: A high source of a particular nutrient must provide at least 20 percent of the daily value.

Exception to the Rule: 2 percent milk, although it does not meet the low-fat standards of 3 grams of fat per serving (it contains 5 grams) can still be called low-fat.

Understanding the Other Labels

What does "organic" mean?

Organic is a general term that means that food is grown or processed without the use of pesticides, synthetic fertilizers, fungicides, waxes, or other chemical additives. At one time, organic was used very freely, and some food that was labeled organic may not have actually been chemical-free. In September 1993, the National Organic Standards Law took effect, which required that any food with the organic label meet certain stringent criteria. First, the organic farm has to be monitored by state or private inspectors to make sure that the farming practices and/or processing procedures meet the organic guidelines. The organic food is then certified and shipped to stores or distributors in specially numbered cartons. Consumers can then ask their green-grocers or supermarket managers to see the certification to verify the authenticity of the product.

Organic doesn't necessarily mean that a food is 100 percent chemical-free. Chemical contamination can occur in many different ways: fertilizers can seep into the soil by irrigation water, or pesticides can be carried from field to field by the wind. However, organic produce has far fewer chemicals than regular produce, and is not deliberately waxed or sprayed. It's somewhat more expensive, but I feel that it's well worth the price.

What does a kosher label mean?

Kosher food is usually designated by a U or a K, often with a D for dairy or an M for meat. Kosher certification has nothing to do with nutrition, or cleanliness for that matter; it merely means that the food has been handled or processed according to the Jewish dietary laws as prescribed in the Book of Leviticus, in the Old Testament. Kosher dietary laws prohibit the consumption of pork and shellfish and the mixing of milk and meat during a meal. Only animals without split hooves and who chew their cuds, like cows and sheep, are kosher. Animals with split hooves, like pigs, are not kosher. Some of these laws may reflect health concerns—the ban on pork could have originated from a fear of trichinosis. Others do not seem to have a health-related background. For instance, according to Orthodox Jewish law, utensils that are used with milk are not to be used with meat, and vice versa. This ban is based on spiritual, as opposed to nutritional, concerns.

Foods that are designated as "Kosher-D" (dairy) are cooked separately from meat or meat products. In order to be labeled kosher, meat and poultry must be slaughtered in a certain way, and only certain cuts of meat can be used. Meat inspectors check for any blemishes and for other signs of disease and deformity. An animal that is sick or shows signs of illness is not considered kosher. Chicken and meat are routinely salted, which may kill some bacteria. However, this extra sodium can pose a threat to people with high blood pressure.

People who are allergic to milk or shellfish may find the kosher label useful if they want to avoid these products. To avoid milk products, simply buy kosher food with an M or a label that states it is not designated as a dairy food.

CHAPTER 14

The Food Irradiation Story

The term "food irradiation" conjures up the image of radioactive, glow-in-the-dark entrées; but in reality, irradiated food looks just like other food, and frankly that's precisely what has me worried.

In the irradiation process, food is bombarded with low levels of radioactivity emitted from a radioactive isotope. The purpose is to kill bacteria, fungi, insects, and many other undesirable creatures that may spread disease. The food does not become radioactive; however, irradiation can cause other changes in the molecular structure of food, notably an increase in free radicals (the unstable molecules that can cause normal cells to mutate) and the formation of other potentially carcinogenic chemicals. Although as proponents of irradiation point out, carcinogens occur naturally in many foods, I feel that it's crazy to go out of your way to increase the quantity of carcinogens in your diet.

In addition, the proliferation of food-irradiation plants throughout the country may pose a hazard for the communities that house these plants. The same issues that plague nuclear power plants, such as the disposal of nuclear waste and worker safety, are also relevant in the debate over irradiation.

There is also evidence that irradiation may significantly reduce the vitamin content of many foods. In fact, one Japanese study showed that irradiated potatoes had lost roughly 50 percent of their vitamin C content, and that irradiated chicken breasts lost about 9 percent of their thiamine content.

The goals of food irradiation—maintaining a safe food supply—are lofty ones. The government estimates that about six million people become ill from food poisoning each year,

although some consumer groups contend that the number is actually much higher. About 9000 people will actually die from eating tainted food. For example, in 1992, hamburgers tainted with the deadly *E. coli* 0157:H7 bacterium were responsible for the deaths of several children in the United States. Irradiation can destroy this bacterium; however, so can proper cooking, as long as the meat is cooked at high enough temperatures. In fact, careful sanitary procedures—

well-inspected and well-run meat-processing plants—can go a long way in preventing problems such as *E. coli* from occurring in the first place. (This is especially true for *E. coli,* which is typically caused by fecal contamination of meat.)

Whether or not food is irradiated, food safety is still a major problem. Irradiation does not kill all bacteria, and food can become tainted after it is irradiated if it is not handled in a safe and wholesome manner.

To add to the debate against irradiation, there have been very few studies on the long-term effects of a steady diet of irradiated food on humans. We simply don't know whether irradiation will prove to be harmful ten or twenty years down the road. For all of these reasons, I feel that irradiation is not a good idea. However, it appears that the USDA is going to allow irradiation; therefore, consumers are going to have to take steps to protect themselves.

First, many states have already banned the sale of irradiated food, and if you live in one of these, you can rest assured that the food in your stores has not been irradiated. If you don't, you have to be vigilant about what you buy. Current regulations require that irradiated food carry a "radura" symbol (a benign-looking flower within a broken circle) to let consumers know that the food has been specially processed. If it's got the symbol, simply don't buy it. However, you can't be sure whether the food you get in restaurants or an ingredient in processed foods has been irradiated. Therefore, consumers need to urge restaurant owners and food manufacturers to avoid using irradiated products. As of this writing, several major companies have already agreed not to irradiate their food, due to public pressure.

Foods for Life

...

CHAPTER 15

The New Vegetarians

When I was growing up in Canada, vegetarians were considered to be quite eccentric. Today, however, vegetarianism is quite commonplace. In fact, according to the *Wellness Letter,* published by the University of California at Berkeley, about 5 percent of Americans, 12 million people, claim to be vegetarians.

It's not difficult to understand why so many people are attracted to a vegetarian diet. Some people may reject meat for religious or moral reasons (such as the Seventh-Day Adventists), but many others have their own best interest at heart. The vegetarian diet is basically a healthy one: It is high in fruit, vegetables, and fiber and relatively low in fat, especially saturated fat. In fact, several studies have shown that vegetarians live longer, have lower blood pressure and lower cholesterol levels, and suffer from fewer diseases than people who eat a diet rich in meat. For example, a recent study in Germany noted that people who follow even a modified vegetarian diet—that is, eat meat only rarely— suffer only one-third the rate of heart disease and about half the rate of cancer as the general population. In addition, there's good evidence that a vegetarian diet can be therapeutic. In his book *Dr. Dean Ornish's Program for Reversing Heart Disease,* Dr. Ornish prescribes a vegetarian diet for heart patients, along with exercise and stress management techniques. Based on Dr. Ornish's studies, patients showed dramatic improvements within a year's time, and were in better shape than many patients who had undergone surgery or who were heavily medicated.

There are many different styles of vegetarianism: The following section outlines the major types.

- Vegans avoid all food of animal origin, including dairy products.
- Lactovegetarians eat dairy products along with plant food (fruits, vegetables, and grains).
- Ovolactovegetarians eat eggs in addition to dairy products and plant food.
- Pescovegetarians add fish to the menu, in addition to dairy and plant food (and sometimes eggs).
- Quasi vegetarians may eat small quantities of chicken and fish in addition to dairy and eggs. Usually, quasi vegetarians don't eat red meat (although I know a few who may give in to the urge to eat a steak once or twice a year).

Although vegetarianism is basically sound and healthy, vegetarians have to make sure that they are getting enough vitamins, minerals, and nutrients. In particular, parents who have their children on a vegetarian regime must take special pains to ensure that their children are getting a well-rounded diet.

Protein: The Right Kind and the Right Amount

Surprisingly, getting enough protein is not a problem for most vegetarians, even though meat is a major source of protein in the American diet. In reality, most Americans get roughly twice as much protein as they actually need. (The RDA is 50 grams of protein daily; however, many Americans consume more than 100 grams.) In fact, many experts believe that even 50 grams of protein is excessive; they cite studies that show that a high-protein diet may be linked to a higher incidence of cancer.

However, no one disputes the fact that the right amount of protein is important for the normal growth and maintenance of body tissues. Protein is composed of smaller units called amino acids, which combine in different ways to form various cells and tissues in the body. There are twenty-two different amino acids: fourteen of these can be made by the body, and the eight others, called essential amino acids, must be obtained through food. (The eight essential amino acids are isoleucine, leucine, lysine, methionine, phenylalanine, threonine, tryptophan, and valine. A ninth amino acid, histidine, is essential for infants and children.)

Animal products—meat, eggs, and dairy—have proteins that contain all eight of these essential amino acids, in addition to some others. Plant food typically does not contain all eight essential amino acids (with the exception of the protein found in soybeans, soy milk, and a handful of grains.) Obviously, lactovegetarians and ovolactovegetarians—people who eat dairy or dairy plus eggs—are able to easily meet their quota of essential amino acids. Vegans, who avoid all animal products, may have a tougher time.

However, this problem can be overcome by different combinations of plant food. For example, the essential amino acids that are missing in grains are present in legumes; therefore, a dish of rice and beans, a meal of baked beans and whole grain bread, or a peanut butter sandwich would provide all eight essential amino acids. When two different foods combine to provide the eight essential amino acids, they are called *complementing* proteins.

At one time, it was believed that complementing proteins had to be eaten together for them to work; however, now we know that as long as you consume enough complementing proteins within the course of a day, you will end up with a complete protein.

Vitamin B_{12}

Vitamin B_{12} is essential for the formation of red blood cells and is necessary for the proper utilization of folic acid. B_{12} deficiency can result in pernicious anemia, a potentially life-threatening problem. As vitamins go, B_{12} is an important one, and unfortunately is found only in foods of animal origin (meat, fish, eggs, and dairy). One study showed that signs of B_{12} deficiency were evident in breast-fed children of mothers who are vegans. Therefore, vegetarians who do not eat any animal food—especially nursing mothers—should take a B_{12} supplement. (The RDA is 2 mcg.)

Calcium

There is concern that people who avoid dairy foods will not get enough of this bone-building mineral. However, calcium is present in foods other than dairy products. For example, green leafy vegetables (such as kale and broccoli), calcium-fortified cereal and orange juice, calcium-enriched tofu, tortillas, and sunflower seeds are reasonably good sources of calcium. Interestingly enough, studies show that plant eaters do not have a higher rate of osteoporosis than lactovegetarians or ovolactovegetarians. In fact, some studies suggest that excessive protein may inhibit the absorption of calcium by the body, so even though plant eaters may not be getting the same quantity of calcium as nonplant eaters, they may be better able to absorb the calcium that they are getting.

Iron

Iron is another mineral that is found in abundance in meat and in smaller quantities in plant food. Studies show that women vegetarians in particular had low levels of serum ferritin (iron stores) in the body, which could result in anemia. Therefore, menstruating girls and women on vegetarian regimes should be careful to include high-iron foods in their diet. Good nonmeat sources of iron include dried fruit, iron-fortified cereals, pumpkin seeds, and sesame seeds. Iron is better absorbed if eaten with a good source of vitamin C, such as orange or tomato.

Zinc

Vegetarians who don't eat eggs or seafood may fall short of this mineral. Although zinc is present in some plant food, it is in a form that is more difficult to absorb than the zinc from animal food. Yeast-leavened whole grain products may help in zinc absorption by blocking the action of zinc inhibitors. Good vegetarian sources of zinc include dried beans, lentils, and nuts and seeds.

Complementing Proteins

The following list shows how meals can be planned around complementing proteins to form complete proteins:

♦ Whole wheat pasta, sautéed with pine nuts (and also vegetables). Lactovegetarians can add a sprinkle of Parmesan cheese.
♦ Meatless chili (sin carne) and brown rice.
♦ Tortilla with beans. Lactovegetarians can add a grated low-fat Cheddar or Monterey Jack for extra flavor.
♦ Cashew butter on whole grain bread.
♦ Eggplant parmigiana made with low-fat cheese, or tofu cheese substitute.

CHAPTER 16

The Hot Foreign Cuisines

As Americans move away from their standard "meat and potatoes" fare, they are learning about other culinary traditions from all across the world. The following section reviews some of the healthiest foreign cuisines and how to make them work for you.

The Mediterranean Diet

Mediterranean countries have a substantially lower rate of heart disease than the United States. Thus, many researchers believe that the Mediterranean diet may offer some protection against heart attack, stroke, and other forms of cardiovascular disease as well as certain forms of cancer.

It's not that the Mediterranean diet is particularly low in fat. In fact, it is as high in fat as the standard American diet, or even higher. For example, the typical Italian consumes between 35 to 40 percent of his daily calories in the form of fat (as compared with 37 percent in the United States). However, unlike in the United States, the fat of choice is olive oil. Saturated fats (such as butter and lard) and other forms of polyunsaturated fats (such as corn oil and safflower oil) are conspicuously absent from Italian kitchens. (The same is true in other Mediterranean countries, such as Spain, Greece, Turkey, Syria, Lebanon, Egypt, and Morocco.)

Many studies have shown that olive oil can raise HDLs, the "good" cholesterol, and lower LDLs, the "bad" cholesterol. But man (or woman) cannot live on olive oil alone, and I believe that there are other equally important reasons why the Mediterranean diet yields such positive results.

- ♦ Mediterranean cuisine is rich in grains, legumes, fresh fruits and vegetables. Grains and legumes are a terrific source of fiber, which may protect against colon cancer. Fresh fruits and vegetables are loaded with fiber, as well as beta-carotene, vitamin C, and other important plant chemicals that may protect against both heart disease and cancer.

- ♦ The Mediterranean diet is short on processed foods, which may be packed with preservatives and saturated fat and stripped of fiber and nutrients.

- ♦ Meat, which is loaded with saturated fat, is used sparingly.

- ♦ Eggplant, tomato, pepper, garlic, and onions are dietary staples—interestingly enough, these are all foods that are currently being investigated by the National Cancer Institute for potential cancer-fighting properties.

- ♦ The Mediterranean diet also calls for an abundance of herbs and spices, such as rosemary, thyme, sage, and cumin. Many of these herbs and spices are potent antioxidants, which may help protect against atherosclerosis by preventing the oxidation of LDL cholesterol, which is believed to be a major factor in the formation of plaque. (Plaque deposits on the arterial wall can prevent the flow of blood to vital organs, including the heart.)

♦ In many Mediterranean countries, dinner is washed down with a glass of red wine. Red wine contains resveratrol, a substance that appears to lower cholesterol.

PERSONAL ADVICE The Mediterranean diet is not perfect—if you're not careful it's still possible to eat too much of the wrong foods, such as pasta drowned in cream sauce or huge chunks of cheese. However, even though people in the Mediterranean region may enjoy an occasional fettucine Alfredo or end dinner with a slice of Brie, they tend to watch portion size. The average serving of pasta is 3 to 4 ounces, dessert consists of a sliver of cheese and is accompanied by a large piece of fruit. If you want to adapt the Mediterranean diet, be sure that you don't overindulge, or merely substitute one form of saturated fat (meat) for another (cheese).

Asian Cuisines

Until recently, Chinese food was the predominant Asian cuisine in the United States. Today, however, there are many different Asian cuisines to choose from, and each offers something unique in terms of flavor and health.

Chinese

I doubt that there's a town in the United States that doesn't have at least one Chinese restaurant. I've been on streets in

New York where there are two or three on the same block. For people looking for fast and easy carry-out meals, Chinese cuisine can offer a healthy alternative to typical fast food. For the more adventurous who like to cook, Chinese cuisine is relatively easy to prepare and cooks quickly.

Chinese chefs rely heavily on vegetables and rice, and use meat, fish, or fowl only as a condiment. In fact, a typical Chinese dish contains roughly one-fourth the amount of meat normally used in a Western meal. There are other important differences between the Chinese diet and the Western diet.

- The Chinese diet is usually high in fiber and low in fat.
- The Chinese do not use dairy products, which are a major source of saturated fat in the U.S. diet.
- Processed foods and refined sugary sweets are a rarity.
- The Chinese rely on stir-frying (usually in a wok), which cooks food quickly without losing too much of important vitamins.

Several ingredients commonly used in the Chinese diet are known protectors against cancer and heart disease. Chinese cuisine is abundant in vegetables, including a great deal of cruciferous vegetables, such as bok choy (cabbage), cauliflower, and broccoli. These foods are rich in beta-carotene, vitamin C, and other important vitamins and minerals. Szechuan cuisine, known for its "hot" taste, uses chili peppers, which, among other things, can clear nasal congestion, lower cholesterol, and help reduce the inflammation of arthritis.

Herbs and spices, such as ginger, onion, parsley, and garlic, which are commonly used in many dishes, may protect against cardiovascular disease and/or cancer.

PERSONAL ADVICE   Chinese cuisine cooked the right way can be terrific; cooked the wrong way it can be high in fat and salt. Wok cooking is fine, as long as you use as little oil as possible (you can prevent sticking by adding a low-sodium chicken broth). If dining out, avoid the heavily fried dishes such as fried spring rolls or egg rolls (which absorb a great deal of fat) and deep-fried, batter-coated meats and vegetables. Stick to steamed vegetables whenever possible. Order steamed dumplings, hot and sour soup, or cold noodles in sesame sauce for an appetizer; pass on the fatty spare ribs. Do not add soy sauce to your food; it is very high in sodium. Ask for your dishes to be prepared without MSG, a commonly used additive that can cause nausea, headaches, and dizziness in some people. Also, avoid pickled vegetables—they may be carcinogenic.

Japanese

Although second to Chinese, Japanese cuisine is growing in popularity. Similar to Chinese, it is high in vegetables and uses meat, chicken, and fish very sparingly. However, it also uses a good deal of soy products (even more so than Chinese) and may not be suitable for someone on a low-sodium diet (unless, of course, you cook it yourself and modify the recipes).

There are some very good reasons to eat a Japanese-style diet. Here are some of them:

♦ Women in Japan have much lower rates of breast cancer, and men have lower rates of prostate cancer, than women or men in the United States. Soy products (soybeans, miso, and tofu), which are high in hormonelike compounds, may protect against these forms of cancer.

- ◆ The Japanese diet is rich in seafood, especially fish such as tuna and salmon, which are high in omega-3 fatty acids. Omega-3 fatty acids protect against heart disease and various forms of cancer.
- ◆ The mushrooms used in Japanese cooking (reishi and shiitake) may protect against cancer and may lower cholesterol, which protects against heart disease.
- ◆ Seaweed, which is commonly used in sushi and other dishes, is a good source of B vitamins and antioxidant vitamins C and E.
- ◆ Green tea, the traditional Japanese tea, may help prevent cavities, lower cholesterol, and prevent the kind of oxidative damage to cells that can cause cancer.

PERSONAL ADVICE　Avoid tempura or battered fried foods; they're very high in fat. Stick with broiled or steamed dishes that are made with very little added fat. If you eat sashimi (raw fish) or sushi, raw fish wrapped in rice and seaweed, keep in mind that raw fish can contain parasites and bacteria. Make sure that the restaurant does a high-volume business and inspects the fish thoroughly. The fish should be refrigerated at all times and look fresh. Ask the restaurant owner how often they buy their fish, and what they do with their leftovers. For additional vitamins and fiber, ask for brown rice.

Thai

This is one of my personal favorites, and I'm glad to see that it is catching on throughout the United States. Although it's similar to other Oriental cuisines in that it is high in vegetables and low in meat, Thai cuisine has a taste all its own.

Special ingredients such as Thai eggplant, Kaffir lime, and Thai papaya combine with bamboo shoots, miniature corn, and straw mushrooms to create uniquely Thai dishes that are both healthy and delicious. In addition:

♦ Thai chefs use a lot of wonderful herbs and spices such as coriander, basil, dill, and ginger. Many of these herbs and spices—used for centuries as folk remedies for a wide variety of ailments—are now being examined for potential cancer-fighting properties by serious researchers throughout the world.

♦ Lemon grass (also called citronella) is used in many Thai dishes. Recent studies show that lemon grass oil may help to lower cholesterol.

♦ Many Thai dishes are steamed, which uses very little fat and helps to retain their vitamins.

♦ Thai chefs use a lot of peanut-based sauces, which, although they are high in fat, appear to have a beneficial effect on cholesterol.

PERSONAL ADVICE Many Thai dishes are made with coconut milk, which is relatively high in fat and calories—eat them sparingly. Instead, opt for sauces made from broth or order steamed dishes. Do order beef or chicken sa-tah, skewers of grilled beef or chicken with a peanut-based dipping sauce, but go light on the sauce. (Peanuts may lower cholesterol, but they are high in calories—a little definitely goes a long way.)

Vietnamese

Vietnamese cuisine was introduced into the United States during the early 1970s by the Vietnamese fleeing the fall of

South Vietnam. Vietnamese food is delicately flavored and lighter than many other Asian cuisines.

♦ Vietnamese chefs rarely fry—steaming is the usual mode of cooking.
♦ Meat is rarely used—poultry and seafood are used as condiments in noodle and vegetable dishes.
♦ Vietnamese cuisine uses lots of raw vegetables and salads.
♦ Foods are seasoned with fresh herbs.

PERSONAL ADVICE Try a bowl of "pho" or noodle soup with fresh vegetables, rice noodles, and sliced beef or chicken. It's low in fat, low in calories, and high in taste.

Indian

A unique blend of herbs, spices, and seasonings gives Indian cuisine its distinctive flavor. Since many Hindus do not eat beef (and some are strict vegetarians), many Indian meals are based around alternative, low-fat, high-fiber forms of protein such as lentils, chickpeas, and kidney beans combined with rice or some other grain. Among meat eaters, lamb and chicken are popular, although the portions of meat are relatively small. Curry, a mixture of spices commonly used in Indian cooking on meats and vegetables, may offer many health benefits.

♦ Many curry spices—turmeric (which gives it its yellow color), garlic, and cumin, to name but a few—may have antioxidant properties, which means that they prevent the oxidation of normal cells by free radicals. This helps prevent cancer and heart disease.

- Studies show that curry spices may lower cholesterol and prevent the formation of blood clots.
- Turmeric and cinnamon, two curry spices, enhance the ability of insulin to metabolize glucose, which may help to control diabetes.

There are other healthy reasons to eat Indian food even if curry is not to your taste. Indian chefs use many different vegetables, ranging from green peas to spinach to eggplant, which are all excellent sources of vitamins and fiber. Meats are usually roasted, not fried. Condiments such as yogurt-based or mint-flavored dips and chutney are low in fat.

PERSONAL ADVICE As good as Indian food can be, some dishes should be avoided, especially if you're watching your fat intake. For example, deep-fried foods such as poori, the puffy bread, and samosas, vegetable-filled dumplings, are high in fat. There are many different Indian breads to choose from, including chapati, which is cooked on charcoal, and naan, a flat bread that is cooked in a hot clay oven known as a tandoor. Instead of samosas, order a vegetable pullao, a rice and vegetable dish (which is low fat but just as satisfying), or a curried vegetable dish, such as curried cauliflower.

Chicken tandoor—skinless chicken cooked in a yogurt sauce—is a terrific low-fat entrée.

Stay away from ghee, a rich, clarified butter sauce which is used to dip bread and appetizers—it's actually higher in saturated fat than plain butter.

South of the Border

Mexican food is one of the most popular foreign cuisines in the United States. Unfortunately, many restaurants (especially fast-food chains) have managed to corrupt this basically healthy cuisine by adding mounds of fatty cheese, sour cream, and meat to what is basically low-fat, healthy fare. This doesn't mean that you should avoid Mexican restaurants, just order wisely. Here are some things that you should keep in mind.

- True Mexican cuisine relies heavily on combining legumes and grains to provide low-cost sources of protein (the so-called Mexican peasant diet). Rice and beans or tortilla (made from cornmeal) and beans are a typical dish. Meat is used sparingly, if at all. (Avoid refried beans; they're often cooked with lard, which is high in saturated fat.)

- Mexican dishes are routinely seasoned with a wide variety of spices, including coriander, cumin, oregano, parsley, garlic, and, of course, chili peppers. All of these foods and herbs are considered potential weapons against heart disease and cancer.

- Salsa, chopped salad usually made from tomatoes, chilies, and onion, is practically the national dish of Mexico. It is a wonderful way to add flavor without adding salt or fat (other than the sodium from the tomato).

- Mexican chefs often combine seafood with vegetables and beans to form a soup or stew, which is a sensible way to reduce the amount of animal protein and fat.

- Fresh fruits and vegetables are dietary staples, especially among the Indian population. Tomatoes, potatoes (all varieties), avocados, squash, and papaya are popular and are all excellent sources of vitamins and nutrients.

- If you order a dish that comes with cheese, such as tacos, ask that the chef use half the amount.

- Beware the tempting basket of tortilla chips on the table. These chips are high in fat and sodium.

- Guacamole, a dip made from avocado, can be laden with mayonnaise, which is high in fat. Salsa is a good substitute.

CHAPTER 17

A Guide to Grains

At one time in the United States, people who couldn't afford meat were forced to "make do" by eating grains. As Americans become more concerned about reducing their rate of cancer and heart disease, grains are no longer regarded as poor man's fare; they are becoming the food of choice. An excellent source of fiber and vitamins, and low in fat, grains are growing in popularity by leaps and bounds. The following list reviews some of the "hot" grains that are being rediscovered by a new generation of health-conscious consumers.

Amaranth

This grain, once a dietary staple of the Aztec Indians, is a small seed that resembles millet and can be eaten as a cereal or side dish. Amaranth is rich in lysine, an amino acid missing from most grains, and is high in calcium and iron. Various amaranth products (such as flakes) are being sold in health food stores; many contain very little amaranth. Buy the real stuff and cook it yourself—it's not any more difficult than making rice, and well worth the effort.

Barley

This ancient grain dates back to the Stone Age as evidenced by fragments of barley and wheat cakes uncovered by archaeologists. Barley is a good source of plant protein, and is rich in B vitamins and both soluble and insoluble fiber. (Soluble fiber lowers cholesterol, and insoluble promotes bowel regularity.) Most supermarkets carry pearled barley, a heavily processed version of this grain, the bran of which is removed and vitamins and minerals are added back. If you shop in health food stores, you will find forms of this grain that you may not find in your local supermarket, such as whole hulled barley, only the outer husk of which is removed, or Scotch barley, the husk and bran of which are removed and the barley is then coarsely ground. Although these less-processed forms may take longer to cook, they are higher in fiber and, in my opinion, healthier all around.

Bran

Bran refers to the outermost part of the grain that is often lost in processing. Bran is an excellent source of protein, fiber, B vitamins, and minerals.

Brown Rice

Brown rice consists of the husk, bran, and germ of the rice. This grain is a good source of fiber, B vitamins, protein, and minerals and other vitamins. Brown rice makes a good side dish, but I also recommend it for breakfast mixed with a little yogurt or low-fat milk and raisins.

Buckwheat

This grain is actually a fruit of the *Fagopyrum* genus (related to rhubarb). The roasted kernel is called kasha, a traditional eastern European dish. Kasha, which has a nutlike flavor, can be cooked up as a cereal or side dish. Unroasted or white buckwheat has a similar flavor and can be used in similar ways. Buckwheat, an excellent source of fiber, has small amounts of vitamin E and B vitamins. As grains go, it is an excellent source of protein, and even contains lysine, an essential amino acid missing from most plant food. Buckwheat (kasha) can be found in most supermarkets.

PERSONAL ADVICE Since buckwheat is actually wheat-free, it is good for people with wheat allergies.

Bulgur

Bulgur is wheat that has been steamed and dried before being ground. A traditional Middle Eastern grain, bulgur makes a terrific side dish, and is used in pilafs and tabouli. It is high in fiber, potassium, and B vitamins.

Couscous

Couscous is made from granular semolina wheat and is a good source of fiber, B vitamins, and iron. Although there are packaged instant forms of this grain on the market, I don't recommend them (they're a lot like eating paste). Buy the real stuff at the health food store. Couscous should be steamed in a special couscousiere, a special pot with a built-in colander, or in a heavy pot in which you can place your own colander. (Line it with cheesecloth to prevent seepage.) Cooking time is about an hour. Serve couscous warm as a side dish (add a handful of cashews, almonds, or dried fruit) or cold mixed with vegetables as a pasta salad.

Cracked Rye

Whole rye kernels cook up to make a delicious breakfast cereal with a good dose of B vitamins and fiber. Top with fresh fruit, fruit preserves, or brown sugar. Rye kernels are available at many health food stores.

Creamed Cereals

Despite their name, creamed cereals do not contain cream; rather they are whole grain flours mixed with water and cooked. Cream of wheat and cream of rice are two popular cream cereals that are widely available in supermarkets. I prefer to use cream cereals that are made from whole grain flour because they are higher in fiber and vitamins.

Granola

Granola cereal is usually made from oats, plus a bunch of other delicious things such as nuts, dried fruit, and seeds. Sweeteners such as honey or molasses are often added. On the positive side, granola is high in fiber, B vitamins, potassium, and vitamin E. The downside is that many commercial granolas are very high in sugar and fat, and should be avoided. There are some newer granolas on the market, however, that contain less than 2 grams of fat per serving—and even a no-fat variety—and are quite tasty.

Grits

Grits doesn't refer to a particular type of grain, rather to how the grain is processed. When a grain is cracked to reduce cooking time, it is called grits. Grits can be made from corn, barley, brown rice, and soy. Corn grits, the most common variety, can be found in many supermarkets. In the South, grits are served as a side dish with breakfast.

PERSONAL ADVICE   Stone-ground grits, which can be found in many health food stores, are far superior to the instant stripped-down version found in supermarkets. They are higher in fiber and vitamins, and taste a lot better too.

Kamut

Kamut, also known as *Triticum polonicum,* is related to the wheat family and has been used since ancient times. It is reputed to be easier to digest than wheat, and can supposedly be better tolerated by people with wheat sensitivity. Kamut cereal is available in health food stores.

Oatmeal

Oatmeal contains oat bran, which has been shown to lower blood cholesterol levels. It is high in fiber, low in fat, and an excellent choice for breakfast. For taste and nutrition, I prefer the old-fashioned long-cooking variety, which you can buy at most health food stores. Sweeten to taste with raisins (for added iron and potassium) or brown sugar.

Quinoa

Pronounced "keen-wa," this "grain" is actually the fruit of an herb that is native to the Andes. Quinoa is rich in all eight essential amino acids, which makes it a complete protein. It is packed with potassium and iron and contains some zinc and B vitamins. Quinoa has a mild flavor, and can be used as a side dish with beans or meat.

Spelt

Spelt is related to the wheat family and, similar to kamut, is reputed to be more easily tolerated by wheat-sensitive people. Spelt is high in fiber and rich in B vitamins. It is a good source of protein and contains all eight of the essential amino acids usually missing in nonanimal foods.

Triticale

This has the distinction of being the first man-made grain, and is actually a hybrid of wheat and rye. It is higher in protein than either wheat or rye, and is rich in lysine, an essential amino acid often lacking in grains. Triticale flour, whole triticale berries, and flaked triticale are available at many health food stores. (You probably won't find this one at the supermarket, yet.) Follow the cooking directions on the package. In some cases, triticale flakes may substitute for oats in certain recipes.

Resources

Throughout *Food as Medicine,* I recommend working with a medical practitioner who is knowledgeable in nutrition. The following is a list of organizations that can help you locate medical professionals in your area or can provide information on nutrition.

(It should be understood that no endorsement or other opinion of any practitioner contacted through these services should be inferred.)

To find a medical practitioner, contact:

American Holistic Medical Association
2002 Eastlake Avenue East
Seattle, WA 98102
(206) 322-6842

American Association of Naturopathic Physicians
P.O. Box 20386
Seattle, WA 98102
(206) 323-7610

Naturopathic physicians are graduates of a four-year postgraduate program in the basic medical sciences. Their training also includes courses in nutrition and herbal medicine. Although they must pass a state licensing examination, naturopathic physicians are allowed to diagnose and treat patients in only ten states. In other states, a naturopathic physician may work under the supervision of an M.D.

American Academy of Environmental Medicine
P.O. Box 16106
Denver, CO 80216
(303) 622-9755

American Holistic Nurses' Association
Box 116
Telluride, CO 81435

For information on finding a qualified nutrition counselor, contact:

The American Dietetic Association
216 W. Jackson
Suite 800
Chicago, IL 60606
(312) 899-0040

For information on cancer and nutrition, contact:

American Institute for Cancer Research
1759 R St., N.W.
Washington, DC 20009
1-800-843-8114

For information on cancer and nutrition, or to locate a chapter of the American Cancer Society in your area, contact:

American Cancer Society
1-800-ACS-2345

For information on diabetes, contact:

American Diabetes Association
1660 Duke Street
Alexandria, VA 22314

For information on fiber research and diabetes, contact:

HCF Nutrition Research Foundation
P.O. Box 22124
Lexington, KY 40522
1-800-727-4423

For information on heart disease, or to find your local chapter of the American Heart Association, contact:

American Heart Association
National Center
7272 Greenville Avenue
Dallas, TX 75231-4596
1-800-242-8721

For information on food safety, contact:

USDA's Meat and Poultry Hotline
1-800-535-4555
(Mon-Fri, 10-4 EST.)
The hotline answers questions on nutrition and food
safety.

For information on flax, contact:

Natural Ovens of Manitowoc
4300 Country Road
Manitowoc, WI 54220
(414) 758-2500

For information about seafood, contact:

The American Seafood Institute's Seafood Hotline
1-800-328-3474

To receive a list of pamphlets offered by the hotline, send a self-addressed, stamped, business-size envelope to:

ASI
406-A Main Street
Wakefield, RI 02879

For information on women's health issues, contact the following groups:

National Women's Health Center
1325 G Street, NW
Washington, DC 20005

American College of Obstetricians and Gynecologists
409 12th Street, SW
Washington, DC 20024-2188
(202) 638-5577

For information on current nutrition news, subscribe to the following newsletters:

Tufts University Diet and Nutrition Letter
P.O. Box 857
Boulder, CO 80322

Environmental Nutrition
2112 Broadway
Suite 200
New York, NY 10023

Nutrition Action Healthletter
Center for Science and the Public Interest
1875 Connecticut Avenue, NW
Suite 300
Washington, DC 20009-5728
(202) 332-9110

Earl Mindell's Healthier Living Newsletter
c/o Phillips Publishing, Corp.
7811 Montrose Road
Potomac, MD 20897-5400
1-800-777-5005

Brief Glossary

The following terms are used frequently throughout this book:

Atherosclerosis: A condition that occurs when arteries become clogged with a thick, waxy substance called plaque, thus impeding the flow of blood to the heart, brain, and other vital organs.

Carcinogen: A cancer-promoting substance.

Cholesterol: A waxy, yellowish, fatlike substance that is produced in the liver and in specialized cells throughout the body. A blood cholesterol level over 200 mg/dl is believed to increase the risk of developing coronary artery disease.

Coronary artery disease: A condition that occurs when the arteries feeding blood to the heart become clogged with plaque, restricting the flow of blood to the heart.

Diastolic blood pressure: Blood pressure is recorded in two numbers. The bottom number, the diastolic pressure, is the pressure in the arteries when the heart muscle relaxes between beats. (See *systolic pressure.*)

DNA (deoxyribonucleic acid): The nucleic acid in chromosomes that controls heredity.

Enzyme: A protein that acts as a catalyst to speed up a chemical reaction in the body.

FDA: Food and Drug Administration.

Free radicals: Highly reactive oxygen molecules that may trigger cancerous changes in cells and may also be responsible for premature aging and atherosclerosis.

GRAS: Generally recognized as safe by the FDA.

Heterocyclic aromatic amines (HAAs): Carcinogenic compounds produced by cooking meat at very high temperatures.

HDL (high-density lipoprotein): Also known as "good cholesterol," HDL carries unused cholesterol to the liver for secretion in bile. A high HDL level is believed to reduce the risk of having a heart attack.

IU: International unit, a measure used for most fat-soluble vitamins.

LDL (low-density lipoprotein): Also known as "bad cholesterol," LDL is the body's major carrier of cholesterol through the blood. A high LDL level may trigger the production of plaque, which can clog arteries bringing blood to the heart and other organs.

Lipids: Lipids are compounds that are not soluble in water. They include fatty acids, steroids, and other important chemicals found in the body.

mg/dl: Milligrams per deciliter.

Nitrites: Used to cure meats, nitrites can combine with chemicals in the stomach to form nitrosamines, which are carcinogenic.

Polycyclic aromatic hydrocarbons (PAHs): These cancer-causing compounds occur when meat is being barbecued over a direct flame, and the fat from the meat drips down into the coals. The carcinogenic fumes then drift up and coat the meat.

RDA: The Recommended Daily Allowance as established by the Food and Nutrition Board of the National Research Council of the Academy of Sciences.

RE: Retinol equivalents, a measure for vitamin A and beta-carotene.

Systolic pressure: Blood pressure is measured by two numbers. The top number measures the systolic pressure, which is generated when the heart contracts and pushes blood into the arteries.

USRDA: U.S. Recommended Daily Allowances were formulated by the FDA to be the legal standards for the nutrient content of food labeling. They are based on the high end of the RDA.

Selected Bibliography

Adlercreutz, H., Honjo, Hideo, Higashi, Akane, et al. "Urinary Excretion of Lignans and Isoflavonoid Phyto-estrogens in Japanese Men and Women Consuming a Traditional Japanese Diet." *American Journal of Clinical Nutrition* 54:1093–1100, 1991.

"Agreements Signed to Test Foods for Cancer Prevention." *Journal of the National Cancer Institute* 83(15):1050–1052, August 7, 1991.

American Cancer Society. "Cancer Facts & Figures—1992."

American Heart Association. "Heart and Stroke Facts," 1993.

American Heart Association. "Liquid Corn Oil May Be Healthier for Heart Than Stick Margarine, Study Suggests," February 19, 1993.

American Heart Association. "Low HDL Cholesterol May Be a Diagnostic Crystal Ball." *Heartstyle* 3 (1):Winter, 1992–93.

American Heart Association. "Search for Best 'Antioxidants' to Protect LDL Points to Vitamin E, New Study Suggests," April 1993.

American Heart Association. "Vitamin E May Help Protect Heart from Effects of Bypass Surgery," November 12, 1990.

American Heart Association. "Vitamins Reduce Risk of Stroke, Heart Disease in Healthy Women," November 13, 1991.

American Institute for Cancer Research. "All About Fat and Cancer Risk." AICR Information Series, 1992.

American Institute for Cancer Research. "Dietary Fiber to Lower Cancer Risk." AICR Information Series, 1992.

American Institute for Cancer Research: "Dietary Guidelines to Lower Cancer Risk." AICR Information Series, 1990.

Anderson, James (ed.). "Beans Are a Blessing." *HCF Nutrition News,* Spring 1992.

Anderson, James. "Be Heart Smart . . . the HCF Way to a Healthy Heart." Lexington, Ky.: HCF Nutrition Research Foundation, 1989.

Anderson, James. "Plant Fiber in Foods." Lexington, Ky.: HCF Nutrition Research Foundation, 1990.

Anderson, James, Gilinsky, Norman H., Deakins, Dee A., et al. "Lipid Responses of Hypercholesterolemic Men to Oat-Bran and Wheat-Bran Intake." American Journal of Clinical Nutrition 54:678–683, 1991.

Anderson, James, Riddell-Mason, Susan, Gustafson, Nancy J., et al. "Cholesterol-Lowering Effects of Psyllium-Enriched Cereal as an Adjunct to a Prudent Diet in the Treatment of Mild to Moderate Hypercholesterolemia." *American Journal of Clinical Nutrition* 56:93–98, 1992.

Aquino, R., Conti, C., De Simone, F., et al. "Antiviral Activity of Constituents of *Tamus communis.*" *Journal of Chemotherapy* 3(5):305–309, October 1991.

Belizan, Jose M., Villar, Jose, Gonzalez, Laura, et al. "Calcium Supplementation to Prevent Hypertensive Disorders of Pregnancy." *New England Journal of Medicine* 325(20): 1399–1404, 1991.

Bennett, Fiona C., and Ingram, David M. "Diet and Female Sex Hormone Concentrations: An Intervention

Study for the Type of Fat Consumed." *American Journal of Clinical Nutrition* 52:808–812, 1990.

Berry, Elliot M., Eisenberg, Shlomo, Friedlander, Yechiel, et al. "Effects of Diets Rich in Monounsaturated Fatty Acids on Plasma Lipoproteins—the Jerusalem Study. II. Monounsaturated Fatty Acids vs. Carbohydrates." *American Journal of Clinical Nutrition* 56:394–403, 1992.

Bitterman, Wilhelm, Farhadian, Haim, Samru, Christine Abu, et al. "Environmental and Nutritional Factors Significantly Associated with Cancer of the Urinary Tract Among Different Ethnic Groups." *Urologic Oncology* 18(3):501–598, August 1991.

Block, Gladys. "Epidemiologic Evidence Regarding Vitamin C and Cancer." *American Journal of Clinical Nutrition* 54:1310S–1314S, 1991.

Blonk, Marion C., Bilo, J.G., Henk, Nauta, Jos, J.P., et al. "Dose-Response Effects of Fish-Oil Supplementation in Healthy Volunteers." *American Journal of Clinical Nutrition* 52:120–127, 1990.

Booth, George C. *The Food and Drink of Mexico.* New York: Dover Publications, 1964.

Braaten, Jan T., Wood, Peter J., Scott, Fraser W., et al. "Oat Gum Lowers Glucose and Insulin After an Oral Glucose Load." *American Journal of Clinical Nutrition* 53:1425–30, 1991.

Bradlow, Leon H., and Michnovicz, Jon. "A New Approach to the Prevention of Breast Cancer." *Proceedings of the Royal Society of Edinburgh,* 95B:77–86, 1989.

Brown, Andrew J., Roberts, David C. K., Pritchard, Janet E., and Truswell, Stewart A. "A Mixed Australian Fish Diet And Fish-Oil Supplementation: Impact on the Plasma Profile of Healthy Men." *American Journal of Clinical Nutrition* 52:825–833, 1990.

Butrum, Ritva R., Clifford, Carolyn K., and Lanza, Elaine. "NCI Dietary Guidelines: Rationale." *American Journal of Clinical Nutrition* 48:888–895, 1988.

Butterworth, C.E., Hatch, Kenneth, Macaluso, Maurizo, et al. "Folate Deficiency and Cervical Dysplasia." *Journal of the American Medical Association* 267(4):530–532, 1992.

Calories & Weight: The USDA Pocket Guide. U.S. Department of Agriculture Human Nutrition Information Service, Agriculture Information Bulletin 364.

Caraguay, Alegria B. "Cancer-Preventive Foods and Ingredients." *Food Technology* 46(4):65–68, 1992.

Carroll, Kenneth K. "Experimental Evidence of Dietary Factors and Hormone-Dependent Cancers." *Cancer Research* 35:3374–3383, 1975.

Carroll, Kenneth K., and Braden, Laura M. "Differing Effects of Dietary Polyunsaturated Vegetable and Fish Oils on Mammary Tumorigenesis in Rats." *Progress in Lipid Research:* 583–585, 1986.

"Cayenne and Cluster Headache." *HerbalGram* 26, 1992.

Cerda, J.J., Robbins, F.L., Burgin, C.W., et al. "The Effects of Grapefruit Pectin on Patients at Risk for Coronary Artery Disease Without Altering Diet or Lifestyle." *Clinical Cardiology* 11(9):589–594, September 1988.

"Cereal Grain Benefits." *Whole Foods,* October 1992.

Childs, Marian T., Kind, B. Irene, and Knopp, Robert H. "Divergent Lipoprotein Responses to Fish Oils with Various Ratios of Eicosapentaenoic Acid and Docosahexaenoic Acid." *American Journal of Clinical Nutrition* 52:632–639, 1990.

"Chili's Hot Chemistry." *Science News* 142:404, December 12, 1992.

Cholesterol: Your Guide to a Healthy Heart (by the Editors of *Consumer Guide*). Lincolnwood, Ill.: Publications International Limited, 1989.

Cobiac, Lynne, Clifton, Peter M., Abbey, Mavis, et al. "Lipid, Lipoprotein, and Hemostatic Effects of Fish vs. Fish-Oil n-3 Fatty Acids in Mildly Hyperlipidemic Males." *American Journal of Clinical Nutrition* 53:1210–1216, 1991.

Coniglio, John G. "How Does Fish Oil Lower Plasma Triglycerides?" *Nutrition Reviews* 50(7):195–196, July 1992.

Crawford, Michael A. "Nutrition: Heart Disease and Cancer. Are Different Diets Necessary?" *Diet and the Prevention of Coronary Heart Disease,* edited by B. Hallgren et al. New York: Raven Press, 1986.

Dausch, J.G., and Nixon, D.W. "Garlic: A Review of Its Relationship to Malignant Disease." *Preventive Medicine* 19(3):346–361, 1990.

Davis, Adelle. *Let's Get Well.* New York: Harcourt, Brace & World, 1965.

"Dietary Fat: No Link to Breast Cancer." *Science News* 142:276, October 24, 1992.

"Dietary Fat Predicts Breast Cancer's Course." *Science News* 143:23, January 9, 1993.

Dorgan, Joanne F., and Schatzkin, Arthur. "Antioxidant Micronutrients in Cancer Prevention." *Nutrition and Cancer* 5(1):43–49, 1991.

Drevon, Christian A. "Marine Oils and Their Effects." *Nutrition Reviews* 50(4):Part II, April 1992.

"Eating to Lower Your High Cholesterol." U.S. Department of Health and Human Services, Public Health Service National Institutes of Health, NIH Publication No. 87-2920, September 1987.

Eden, Alvin N. *Dr. Eden's Healthy Kids: The Essential Diet, Exercise and Nutrition Program.* New York: New American Library, 1987.

Elegbede, J.A., Elson, C.E., Tanner, M.A., et al. "Regression of Rat Primary Mammary Tumors Following Dietary d-Limonene." *Journal of the National Cancer Institute* 76(2):323–325, February 1986.

Flaten, Hugo, Hostmark, Arne T., Kierulf, Peter, et al. "Fish-Oil Concentrate: Effects on Variables Related to Cardiovascular Disease." *American Journal of Clinical Nutrition* 52:300–306, 1990.

"Flax Facts." *Journal of the National Cancer Institute* 83(15):1050–1052, August 7, 1991.

Fod, Gene. *The Benefits of Moderate Drinking: Alcohol, Health & Society.* San Francisco: Wine Appreciation Guild, 1988.

"Folate Supplements Prevent Recurrence of Neural Tube Defects." *Nutrition Reviews* 50(1):22–24, January 1992.

"Folic Acid for Fighting Birth Defects?" *Tufts University Diet and Nutrition Letter* 10(9): November 1992.

Frei, Balz. "Ascorbic Acid Protects Lipids in Human Plasma and Low Density Lipoprotein Against Oxidative Damage." *American Journal of Clinical Nutrition* 54:1113S–1118S, 1991.

Fritsche, Kevin L., and Johnston, Patricia V. "Effect of Dietary a-Linolenic Acid on Growth, Metastasis, Fatty Acid Profile and Prostaglandin Production of Two Murine Mammary Adenocarcinomas." *Journal of Nutrition* 120:1601–1609, 1990.

Fulder, Stephen, and Blackwood, John. *Garlic: Nature's Original Remedy.* Rochester, Vt.: Healing Arts Press, 1991.

Gallagher, John. *Good Health with Vitamins and Minerals: A Complete Guide to a Lifetime of Safe and Effective Use.* New York: Summit Books, 1990.

Garland, Cedric F., Garland, Frank C., and Gorham, Edward. "Can Colon Cancer Incidence and Death Rates Be Reduced with Calcium and Vitamin D?" *American Journal of Clinical Nutrition* 54:193S–201S, 1991.

"Garlic, the Food-aceutical." *University of California at Berkeley Wellness Letter* 8(6), March 1992.

Gillman, Matthew W., Oliveria, Susan A., Moore, Lynn L., and Ellison, Curtis. "Inverse Association of Dietary Calcium with Systolic Pressure in Young Children." *Journal of the American Medical Association* 267(17), 1992.

Goldberg, Jeanne P. "Nutrition and Health Communication: The Message and the Media Over Half a Century." *Nutrition Reviews* 50(3):71–77, March 1992.

Gotto, A., La Rosa, J., et al. "The Cholesterol Facts: A Summary of the Evidence Relating Dietary Fats, Blood Cholesterol, and Coronary Artery Disease." Commissioned by the Task Force on Cholesterol Issues of the American Heart Association, 1989.

Graham, Saxon, Hellman, Rosemary, Marshall, James, et al. "Nutrient Epidemiology of Postmenopausal Breast Cancer in Western New York." *American Journal of Epidemiology* 134:552–566, 1991.

Greene, Bert. *The Grains Cookbook.* New York: Workman Publishing, 1988.

Griffenhagen, George B. "The Materia Medica of Christopher Columbus." *Pharmacy in History* 34(3):131–145, 1992.

Hatton, Daniel, Muntzel, Martin, Absalon, Jeff, et al. "Dietary Calcium and Iron: Effects on Blood Pressure and Hematocrit in Young Spontaneously Hypertensive Rats." *American Journal of Clinical Nutrition* 53:542–546, 1991.

Heimburger, D. C., Alexander, C.B., Birch R., et al. "Improvement in Bronchial Squamous Metaplasia in

Smokers Treated with Folate and Vitamin B_{12}. Report of a Preliminary Randomized, Double-Blind Intervention Trial." *Journal of the American Medical Association* 259(10):1525–1530, 1988.

Hendler, Sheldon Saul. *The Doctors' Vitamin and Mineral Encyclopedia.* New York: Fireside/Simon & Schuster, 1990.

Hendrickson, Audra, and Hendrickson, Jack. *Broccoli & Company.* Pownal, Vt.: Storey Communications, Inc., 1989.

Herrero, Rolando, Potischman, Nancy, Brinton, Louise A., et al. "A Case-Control Study of Nutrient Status and Invasive Cervical Cancer." *American Journal of Epidemiology* 134(11):1335–1345, 1991.

Hilton, Ellen, Isenberg, H.D., Alperstein, P., et al. "Ingestion of Yogurt Containing *Lactobacillus acidophilus* as Prophylaxis for Candidal Vaginitis." *Annals of Internal Medicine* 116(5):353–357, March 1, 1992.

Hocman, Gabriel. "Prevention of Cancer: Vegetables and Plants." *Compendium of Biochemistry Physiology* 93B(2): 201–212, 1989.

Holleb, Arthur, Fink, Diane, and Murphy, George. *American Cancer Society Textbook of Clinical Oncology.* Atlanta: American Cancer Society, 1991.

Hurley, Jayne, and Schmidt, Stephen. "Bread: Pretty Hot Stuff." *Nutrition Action Healthletter,* October 1992.

"Is Our Fish Safe to Eat?" *Consumer Reports,* February 1992.

Jaakkola, K., Lahteenmaki, P., Laakso, J., et al. "Treatment with Antioxidant and Other Nutrients in Combination with Chemotherapy and Irradiation in Patients with Small-Cell Lung Cancer." *Anticancer Research* 12:599–606, 1992.

Jaffrey, Madhur. *Indian Cooking.* New York: Barron's, 1983.

James, W. Philip T., and Ralph, Ann. "Dietary Fats and Cancer." *Nutrition Research* 12(1):S147–S158, 1992.

Jialal, Ishwarlal. "Can Vitamins Slow the Atherosclerotic Process?" American Heart Associations Writers Forum, 1992.

Johnson, Timothy. "The Cholesterol Controversy." *Harvard Medical School Health Letter* 15(2), December 1989.

Jovanovic, Lois, and Subak-Sharpe, Genell J. *Hormones: The Woman's Answerbook.* New York: Fawcett Columbine, 1987.

Karmali, R.A. "Fatty Acids: Inhibition." *American Journal of Clinical Nutrition* 45:225–229, 1987.

Karmali, R.A. "n-3 Fatty Acids and Cancer." *Journal of Internal Medicine* 225 (Supplement 1):197–200, 1989.

Karmali, R.A., Marsh, Jane, and Fuchs, Charles. "Effect of Omega-3 Fatty Acids on Growth of Rat Mammary Tumor." *Journal of the National Cancer Institute* 73(2): 457–461, July 1984.

Kashtan, Hanoch, Stern, Hartley S., Jenkins, David J.A., et al. "Wheat-Bran and Oat-Bran Supplements' Effects on Blood Lipids and Lipoproteins." *American Journal of Clinical Nutrition* 55:976–980, 1992.

Katsouyanni, K., Trichopoulos, D., Xirouchaki, E., et al. "Diet and Breast Cancer: A Case Controlled Study in Greece." *Internal Journal of Cancer* 38:815–820, 1986.

Khan, A., Bryden, N.A., and Polansky, M.M. "Insulin Potentiating Factor and Chromium Content of Selected Foods and Spices." *Biological Trace Element Research* 24(3):183–188, March 1990.

"Kidney Stones: Don't Curb the Calcium." *Science News* 143, March 27, 1993.

Kinsella, John E., Lokesh, B., and Stone, Richard A. "Dietary n-3 Polyunsaturated Fatty Acids and Amelioration of

Cardiovascular Disease: Possible Mechanisms. *American Journal of Clinical Nutrition* 52:1–28, 1990.

Knight, Kathy B., and Keith, Robert E. "Calcium Supplementation on Normotensive and Hypertensive Pregnant Women." *American Journal of Clinical Nutrition,* 55:891–895, 1992.

Lands, William E.M. "Renewed Questions About Polyunsaturated Fatty Acids." *Nutrition Reviews* 44(6):189–195, June 1986.

Legato, Marianne J., and Colman, Carol. *The Female Heart.* New York: Simon & Schuster, 1991.

Leighton, Terrance, Ginther, Charles, and Fluss, Larry. "The Distribution of Quercetin and Quercetin Glycosides in Vegetable Components of the Human Diet." Presented at the Royal Society of Chemistry Conference, England, 1992.

Liebman, Bonnie. "Seafood: Fishing for Omega-3s." *Nutrition Action Healthletter,* November 1992.

Lifespan Plus (by the editors of *Prevention Magazine*). Emmaus, Pa.: Rodale Press, 1990.

Longcope, Christopher. "Relationships of Estrogen to Breast Cancer, and of Diet to Estradiol Metabolism." *Journal of the National Cancer Institute* 82(11), June 6, 1990.

Mata, Pedro, Alvarez-Sala, Luis A., and Rubio, Maria Jose. "Effects of Long-term Monounsaturated- vs. Polyunsaturated-Enriched Diets on Lipoproteins in Healthy Men and Women." *American Journal of Clinical Nutrition* 55:836–850, 1992.

Matkovic, Velimir, Fontana, Darlene, Tominac, Cedomil, et al. "Factors That Influence Peak Bone Mass Formation: A Study of Calcium Balance and the Inheritance of Bone Mass in Adolescent Females." *American Journal of Clinical Nutrition* 52:878–888, 1990.

McCaleb, Rob. "Cranberry Juice Affects Urinary Tract Infections." *HerbalGram* 26:24, 1992.

McCaleb, Rob. "Hot Chili Getting Hotter!" *HerbalGram* 27, 1992.

McCarron, David, Morris, Cynthia, Young, Eric, et al. "Dietary Calcium and Blood Pressure: Modifying Factors in Special Populations." *American Journal of Clinical Nutrition* 54:215S–219S, 1991.

McIntosh, G.H., Whyte, Joanna, McArthur, Rosemary, and Nestel, Paul J. "Barley and Wheat Foods: Influence on Plasma Cholesterol Concentrations in Hypercholesterolemic Men." *American Journal of Clinical Nutrition* 53:1205–1209, 1991.

McKeown-Eyssen, Gail E., and See, Elizabeth Bright. "Dietary Factors in Colon Cancer: International Relationships." *Nutrition and Cancer* 6(3):160–170, 1984.

Menkes, Marilyn S., Comstock, George W., and Vuilleumier, Jean P. "Serum Beta-Carotene, Vitamin A and E, Selenium, and the Risk of Lung Cancer." *New England Journal of Medicine* 315(20):1250–1254, 1983.

Menon, Nirmala K., and Dhopeshwarkar, Govind A. "Essential Fatty Acid Deficiency and Brain Development." *Progress in Lipid Research* 21:309–326, 1982.

Michnovicz, Jon, and Bradlow, Leon H. "Dietary and Pharmacological Control of Estradiol Metabolism in Humans." *Annals of the New York Academy of Sciences,* pp. 291–299, 1990.

Michnovicz, Jon, and Bradlow, H. Leon. "Inductions of Estradiol Metabolism by Dietary Indole-3-Carbinol in Humans." *Journal of the National Cancer Institute* 82(11), June 6, 1990.

Miller, Mark. *The Great Chile Book.* Berkeley, Ca.: Ten Speed Press, 1991.

Mindell, Earl. *Herb Bible*. New York: Simon & Schuster/ Fireside, 1992.

Mindell, Earl. "26 Ways to Lower Cholesterol Naturally." Adanac Management, Inc., 1990.

Mindell, Earl. *Vitamin Bible*. New York: Warner Books, 1992.

Molgaard, J, von Schenck, H., and Ollson, A.G. "Alfalfa Seeds Lower Low Density Lipoprotein Cholesterol and Apolipoprotein B Concentrations in Patients with Type II Hyperlipoproteinemia." *Atherosclerosis* 65(1–2):173–179, May 1987.

Mowrey, Daniel B. *Next Generation Herbal Medicine*. New Canaan, Conn.: Keats Publishing, Inc., 1988.

MRC Vitamin Study Research Group. "Prevention of Neural Tube Defects: Results of the Medical Research Council Vitamin Study." *The Lancet* 338:131–136, July 20, 1991.

National Institutes of Health, National Cancer Institute: "NCI's 5 a Day Program," July 1, 1992.

Need, Allan G., Morris, Howard A., Cleghorn, David B., et al. "Effect of Salt Restriction on Urine Hydroxyproline Excretion in Postmenopausal Women." *Archives of Internal Medicine* 151:757–759, April 1991.

Negri, Eva, La Vecchia, Carlo, Francheschi, Silvia, et al. "Vegetable and Fruit Consumption and Cancer Risk." *International Journal of Cancer* 48:350–354, 1991.

Nelson, Miriam E., Fisher, Elizabeth C., Dilmanian, F. Avraham, et al. "A 1-Year Walking Program and Increased Dietary Calcium in Postmenopausal Women: Effects on Bone." *American Journal of Clinical Nutrition* 53:1304–1311, 1991.

Neuringer, Martha, and Conner, William. "N-3 Fatty Acids in the Brain and Retina: Evidence of the Essentiality." *Nutrition Reviews* 44(9):285–293, 1985.

New York Academy of Sciences. "Beyond Defficiency: New Views on the Function and Health Effects of Vitamins." February 9–12, 1992.

Nomura, Abraham M.Y., Kolonel, Laurence, N., Hankin, Jean H., et al. "Dietary Factors in Cancer of the Lower Urinary Tract." *International Journal of Cancer* 48:199–205, 1991.

Ornish, Dean. *Dr. Dean Ornish's Program for Reversing Heart Disease.* New York: Random House, 1990.

Packer, Lester. "Protective Role of Vitamin E in Biological Systems." *American Journal of Clinical Nutrition* 53: 1050S-1055S, 1991.

Paolisso, Guiseppe, Sgambato, Saverio, and Gambardella, Antonio. "Daily Magnesium Supplements Improve Glucose Handling in Elderly Subjects." *American Journal of Clinical Nutrition* 55:1161–1167, 1992.

Pauling, Linus. "Effect of Ascorbic Acid on Incidence of Spontaneous Mammary Tumors and UV-Light-Induced Skin Tumors in Mice." *American Journal of Clinical Nutrition* 54:1252S-1255S, 1991.

Pauling, Linus. *Vitamin C and the Common Cold.* New York: Bantam Books, 1971.

Peretz, Anne, Neve, Jean, Desmedt, Jacques, Duchateau, Jean, et al. "Lymphocyte Response Is Enhanced by Supplementation of Elderly Subjects with Selenium Enriched Yeast." *American Journal of Clinical Nutrition* 53:1323–1328, 1991.

Peterson, I. "Pectin Helps Fight Cancers Spread." *Science News* 141:180, March 21, 1992.

Peto, R., Doll, R., Buckley, J.D., and Sporn, M.B. "Can Dietary Beta-Carotene Materially Reduce Human Cancer Rates?" *Nature* 290(19):201–208, 1981.

Potischman, Nancy, Herreo, Rolando, Brinton, Louise A., et al. "A Case-Control Study of Nutrient Status and

Invasive Cervical Cancer." *American Journal of Epidemiology* 134(11):1347–1355, 1991.

Potischman, Nancy, McCulloch, Charles E., Byers, Tim, et al. "Breast Cancer and Dietary and Plasma Concentrations of Carotenoids and Vitamin A." *American Journal of Clinical Nutrition* 52:909–915, 1990.

"Preventing Wintertime Bone Loss: Effects of Vitamin D Supplementation in Healthy Postmenopausal Women." *Nutrition Reviews* 50(2):52–54, February 1992.

Prewitt, T. Elaine, Schmeisser, Dale, Bowen, Phyllis E., et al. "Changes in Body Weight, Body Composition, and Energy Intake in Women Fed High- and Low-Fat Diets." *American Journal of Clinical Nutrition* 54:304–310, 1991.

Pryor, William A. "Can Vitamin E Protect Humans Against the Pathological Effects of Ozone in Smog?" *American Journal of Clinical Nutrition* 53:702–722, 1991.

Ratnayake, W.M.N., Behrens, W.A., Fishcher, P.W.F., et al. "Flaxseed: Chemical Stability and Nutritional Properties." *Proceedings of the Flax Institute of the United States Annual Research Conference,* January 30–31, 1992.

Reay, Devon. "A Potpourri of Peppers." *The Herb Quarterly,* No. 38.

Research Briefs, U.S. Department of Agriculture. April–June, 1992. Information on Chromium Research.

Ripsin, Cynthia M., Keenan, Joseph M., Jacond, David R., et al. "Oat Products and Lipid Lowering: A Meta-Analysis." *Journal of the American Medical Association* 267(24): 3317–3325, June 24, 1992.

Risch, Harvey A., Meera, Jain, Choi, N. Won, et al. "Dietary Factors and the Incidence of Cancer of the Stomach." *American Journal of Epidemiology* 122(6):947–956, 1985.

Robertson, James McD., Donner, Allan P., and Trevithick, John R. "A Possible Role for Vitamins C and E in Cataract Prevention." *American Journal of Clinical Nutrition* 53:346–351S, 1991.

Rolls, Barbara J., Pirraglia, Paul A., Jones, Michaelle B., et al. "Effects of Olestra, a Noncaloric Fat Substitute, on Daily Energy and Fat Intakes in Lean Men." *American Journal of Clinical Nutrition* 56:84–92, 1992.

Rolls, Barbara J., and Shide, David J. "The Influence of Dietary Fat and Body Weight." *Nutrition Reviews* 50(10): 283–289, October 1992.

Rose, David P., Goldman, Madeleine, Connolly, Jeanne M., and Strong, Leslie E. "High Fiber Diet Reduces Serum Estrogen Concentrations in Premenopausal Women." *American Journal of Clinical Nutrition* 54:520–525, 1991.

Rosenberg, Irwin H. "Could Food Labels Be Dangerous to Health?" *Nutrition Reviews* 50(10):298–299, October 1992.

Saketkhoo, K., Januszkiewicz, A., and Sackner, M.A. "Effects of Drinking Hot Water, Cold Water, and Chicken Soup on Nasal Mucus Velocity and Nasal Airflow Resistance." *Chest* 74(4):408–410, October 1978.

Schecter, Arnold. "Some Call It Kosher." *In Health*, November 1991.

Schmidt, D.R., and Sobota, A.E. "An Examination of the Anti-Adherence Activity of Cranberry Juice on Urinary and Nonurinary Bacterial Isolates." *Microbios* 55(224–225):173–181, 1988.

Seidelin, Kaj N., Myrup, Bjarne, and Fischer-Hanson, Birgit. "N-3 Fatty Acids in Adipose Tissue and Coronary Artery Disease Are Inversely Related." *American Journal of Clinical Nutrition* 55:1111–1119, 1992.

Shenoy, N.R., and Choughuley, A.S. "Inhibitory Effect of Diet Related Sulfhydryl Compounds on the Formation of Carcinogenic Nitrosamine." *Cancer Letter* 65(3):227–232, August 31, 1992.

Shute, Wilfrid E., and Taub, Harold J. *Vitamin E for Ailing and Healthy Hearts.* New York: Pyramid Books, 1969.

Simone, Charles B. *Cancer & Nutrition.* Garden City Park, N.Y.: Avery Publishing Group, 1992.

Simopoulos, Artermis P. "Omega-3 Fatty Acids in Health and Disease and in Growth and Development." *American Journal of Clinical Nutrition* 54:438–463, 1991.

Slattery, Martha L., Schumacher, Mary C., West, Dee W., et al. "Food Consumption Trends Between Adolescent and Adult Years and Subsequent Risk of Prostate Cancer." *American Journal of Clinical Nutrition* 52:752–757, 1990.

Sobota, A.E. "Inhibition of Bacterial Adherence by Cranberry Juice: Potential Use for the Treatment of Urinary Tract Infections." *Journal of Urology* 131(5):1013–1016, May 1984.

Sokolov, Raymond. "This Is Quinoa." *Natural History,* June 1992.

Stetchell, K.D.R., Borriello, S.P., Gordon, H., et al. "Lignan Formation in Man—Microbial Involvement and Possible Roles in Relation to Cancer." *The Lancet:* 4–7, July 4, 1981.

Stitt, Paul. *Why George Should Eat Broccoli.* Milwaukee: The Dougherty Company, 1990.

Stolzenburg, William. "Garlic Medicine: Cures in Cloves?" *Science News,* September 1990.

Stroh, M. "Inside Broccoli: A Weapon Against Cancer." *Science News* 141:183, March 21, 1992.

"Supplemental Dietary Potassium Reduced the Need for Antihypertensive Drug Therapy." *Nutrition Reviews* 50(5): 144, May 1992.

Surgeon General's Report on Nutrition and Health. U.S. Department of Health and Human Services. Rockin, Ca.: Prima Publishing and Communications, 1988.

Tannenbaum, A. "The Genesis and Growth of Tumors. III. Effects of a High-Fat Diet." *Cancer Research* 2:468–475, 1942.

Thompson, D.S. (editor). *EveryWoman's Health: The Complete Guide to Body and Mind by 15 Women Doctors.* New York: Prentice-Hall Press, 1985.

Thompson, Lillian U., Robb, Paul, Serraino, Maria and Cheung, Felicia. "Mammalian Lignan Production from Various Foods." Journal of Nutrition and Cancer 16:43–52, 1991.

Thun, Michael J., Calle, Eugenia E., Namboodiri, Mohan M., et al. "Risk Factors for Fatal Colon Cancer in a Large Prospective Study." *Journal of the National Cancer Institute* 84(19):1491–1499, October 7, 1992.

Tinker, Lesley F., Schneeman, Barbara O., Davis, Paul A., et al. "Consumption of Prunes as a Source of Dietary Fiber in Men with Mild Hypercholesterolemia." *American Journal of Clinical Nutrition* 53:1259–1265, 1991.

Toufexis, Anastasia. "The New Scoop on Vitamins." *Time,* April 6, 1992.

Tucker, Don M., Penland, James G., and Sandstead, Harold H. "Nutrition Status and Brain Function in Aging." *American Journal of Clinical Nutrition* 52:93–102, 1990.

United States Department of Agriculture, Food Safety and Inspection Service: "FSIS Backgrounder, Nutrition Labeling of Meat and Poultry Products," January 1993.

United States Department of Agriculture, Human Nutrition Information Service: *Nutritive Value of Foods.* Home and Garden Bulletin Number 72.

VanEenwyk, Juliet, Davis, Faith G., and Bowen, Phyllis E. "Dietary and Serum Carotenoids and Cervical Intraepithelial Neoplasia." *Internal Journal of Cancer* 48:34–38, 1991.

"Vitamin D and Psoriasis." *Nutrition Reviews* 50(5):138–141, May 1992.

"Vitamin E Moves on Stage in Cancer Prevention Studies." *Journal of the National Cancer Institute* 84(13), July 1, 1992.

"Vitamin E Supplementation Enhances Immune Response in the Elderly." *Nutrition Reviews* 50(3):85–87, March 1992.

Weiner, Michael A. *Dr. Weiner's Herbal Reference Guidebook: Herbs and Immunity.* San Rafael, Ca.: Quantum Books, 1990.

Wolf, George. "Retinoids and Carotenoids as Inhibitors of Carcinogenesis and Inducers of Cell-Cell Communication." *Nutrition Reviews* 50(9):270–274, 1992.

Wolmarans, Petro, Benadé, Spinnler, A.J., Kotze, Theunis J.vW., et al. "Plasma Lipoprotein Response to Substituting Fish for Red Meat in the Diet." *American Journal of Clinical Nutrition* 53:1171–1176, 1991.

Wotecki, Catherine E., and Thomas, Paul R. (eds.). *Eat for Life: The Food and Nutrition Board's Guide to Reducing Your Risk of Chronic Disease.* Washington, D.C.: National Academy Press, 1992.

"Yet Another Reason to Drink Your Milk." Tufts University Diet & Nutrition Letter 9(11), January 1992.

You, W.C., Blot, W.J., Chang, Y.S., et al. "Allium Vegetables and Reduced Risk of Stomach Cancer." *Journal of the*

National Cancer Institute 81(2):163–164, January 18, 1989.

Ziegler, Regina G. "Vegetables, Fruits and Carotenoids and the Risk of Cancer." *American Journal of Clinical Nutrition* 53:251S–259S, 1991.

Index

Visit
❖ Pocket Books ❖
online at

....

www.SimonSays.com

....

Keep up on the latest new
releases from your favorite
authors, as well as author
appearances, news, chats,
special offers and more.

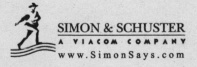

SIMON & SCHUSTER
A VIACOM COMPANY
www.SimonSays.com

Pocket
Books

2381-01